Praise for *Loving to the End … and On*

"The good thing about dying is it opens the door to never-ending love. Lynn Robinson leads us through that door with facts and stories from scientists, physicians, nurses, NDErs, after-death communicators, family members, and the dying themselves. Without sugarcoating what can be painful about navigating the end of life, Lynn guides us through its physical and spiritual process."

—Rev. Terri Daniel, MA, CT, end-of-life advisor, Interfaith Chaplaincy, founder of the Afterlife Awareness Conference

"Death is a natural part of life, but that doesn't make it easy to understand or deal with. As a nurse, I know firsthand the challenges that health-care providers have with caring for patients and families experiencing illness and the uncertainties of health outcomes. Lynn's book provides a perspective on a subject that's often not covered well in the curriculum preparing health professionals. Her insight, experiences, and descriptions garnered through interviews with others help us reframe our perspectives of death and build meaning and hope for those in the helping professions and for their patients. For these reasons, I highly recommend her book."

—Debra C. Davis, PhD, RN, professor of nursing, University of South Alabama

"Lynn Robinson shows some of the many ways that love transforms the death experience. She is at her best when describing examples that point with force to the reality of another world, such as visions of deceased loved ones gathered around the deathbed. Robinson is very much a believer in the world to come and gently invites those who do not share her beliefs to look at the evidence she presents. For her, love begins in this world and continues in the next."

—Stafford Betty, PhD, author of *The After Life Unveiled, When Did You Ever Become Less by Dying? Afterlife: The Evidence*, and *The Severed Breast* (novel)

"In our common human experience, perhaps most dreaded is death. Lynn Robinson offers an antidote for our distress. Only the most hardened or the most hopeless of us would fail to benefit from the messages of those whose stories she tells—unless they choose not to. Along with Lynn, I suggest letting go self-imposed pain. *Loving to the End … and On* will help you do just that, and find peace in the process."

—Paul H. Smith, PhD, Major, US Army, ret., author of *The Essential Guide to Remote Viewing, The Secret Military Remote Perception Skill Anyone Can Learn*

"This book will touch your heart. There truly is no death, and love never, ever dies. Dr. Robinson's book reminds us of those truisms and communicates them in such a gentle and caring way, as it also offers practical advice on moving through a loved one's last days. Whether you already know that there is no death and that our soul goes on or not, you will find many delights in *Loving to the End ... and On*, along with a range of practical information, research, and recommendations. *Loving to the End ... and On: A Guide to the Impossibly Possible* is a gift that will enrich your life—and may open your mind and understanding to more comforting and life-enriching possibilities."

—Diane Brandon, author of *Born Aware: Stories & Insights from Those Spiritually Aware Since Birth, Dream Interpretation for Beginners*, and *Intuition for Beginners*

"Dr. Robinson provides firsthand evidence that love can work almost miraculously in our lives. Using experiences of her own and others, she demonstrates that love expands our sensory capabilities, often breaking conventional time and space boundaries. She recounts visits and messages from those who have died and our own, often unexpected, responses. Love expands our visions and extends our connections with others nearby and far away, in bodies or not. If you have ever been mystified by communications, events, or reactions you may have experienced, Dr. Robinson's interviews and commentary will increase your understanding while focusing on the incredible powers—yes, powers—of love. Love requires exploration and openness. Dr. Robinson's book is certain to open your minds and hearts to experiences and information you might otherwise miss. I highly recommend this book to you."

—John Hadley Strange, PhD, Princeton University

"Having practiced psychiatry for over twenty years, and having known Lynn for all fifty-two of my years of life, I was still surprised and enlightened by Lynn's beautifully written and profoundly insightful book. Lynn teaches us through her direct experiences and observations that life and death are artificial distinctions. People we love die. We die. But we suffer less knowing that death is not the end and that we remain connected in ways that are visible if we foster love and an open mind. I highly recommend her book."

—Gilbert R. Ladd IV, MD, Board-Certified Psychiatrist

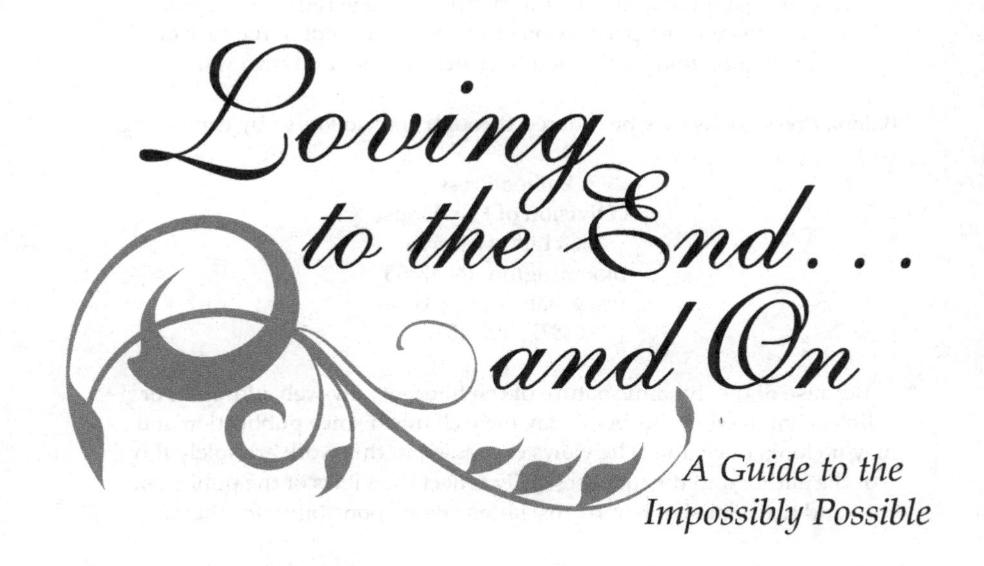

LYNN B. ROBINSON, PH.D.

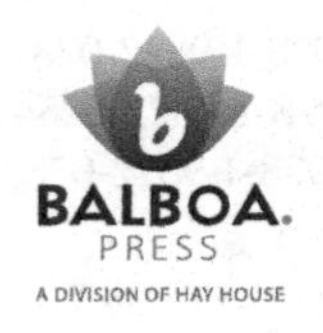

Balboa Press books may be ordered through booksellers or by contacting:

Balboa Press
A Division of Hay House
1663 Liberty Drive
Bloomington, IN 47403
www.balboapress.com
1 (877) 407-4847

Because of the dynamic nature of the Internet, any web addresses or links contained in this book may have changed since publication and may no longer be valid. The views expressed in this work are solely those of the author and do not necessarily reflect the views of the publisher, and the publisher hereby disclaims any responsibility for them.

The author of this book does not dispense medical advice or prescribe the use of any technique as a form of treatment for physical, emotional, or medical problems without the advice of a physician, either directly or indirectly. The intent of the author is only to offer information of a general nature to help you in your quest for emotional and spiritual well-being. In the event you use any of the information in this book for yourself, which is your constitutional right, the author and the publisher assume no responsibility for your actions.

Print information available on the last page.

ISBN: 978-1-9822-0282-8 (sc)
ISBN: 978-1-9822-0284-2 (hc)
ISBN: 978-1-9822-0283-5 (e)

Library of Congress Control Number: 2018905145

Balboa Press rev. date: 05/31/2018

This book is dedicated to you, the reader.
It is also and most lovingly dedicated to Jack, Kathleen, and Susan.

In order to maintain the privacy of the people whose stories were read by me or told to me personally and included in this book, I have used only first names and/or have changed the names.

Contents

Introduction

Thank you for having enough curiosity to read this book. I am truly excited to have you along on this expansive journey into charting new territory for living, learning, and loving each other to the end … and on.

My personal transformative odyssey has stretched across many years. And to be honest, I was not aware of the nature and course of this particular trip or of its destination. My early and insatiable quest to understand consciousness—the nature of being—led me to communicating in ways my rational self said, "no way," which circuitously led to a joyous realization that physical death is the end to only part of who we are. I began sharing with others what I was learning and experiencing.

Though for twenty years I have been encouraged to write another book about possibilities that some skeptics find so threatening they categorically deny them, I've started a few times and abandoned the projects. Until this time.

What is my stimulus for writing now? I had an offer I couldn't refuse. In 2013, a good friend and dean of a college of nursing called to ask me if I would consider teaching an online credit course about near-death experiences. It didn't happen, but not because of me. Instead, the NDE request became the motivation for this book, but neither its lone nor primary orientation.

A more inclusive theme evolved into end-of life care as a pathway for affirming that love is always available, that our loved ones never fully leave us, and that every day can be another day of loving, because physical bodies die, but love does not. Research, reinforced by personal experience, affirmed that some of us already sense that those we love continue in some nonphysical reality; some of us are becoming more open to that possibility; and some of us continue to insist that life begins, ends, and is finite. Preparation and investigation lead to those who share their lives with us, who share their NDEs, their predeath visions, and their after-death communications; it extended bedside to the physical care, and mis-care, of those who are nearing death. And it repeatedly illustrated that the one constant—in whatever form it takes, whether only in memory or in some other way—is love.

And so, the teaching request became a nexus to something more. I had been told that to teach the NDE course, I had to complete certification for using university online protocol. I did that. And while doing that, I did hours and hours of research and writing based on related course offerings in a variety of campus and internet offerings. I created a syllabus for a nursing school program. I won't take you through the numerous administrative hurdles I was asked to jump, just one that I could not—the one that would become the initial backbone of this creation: I could provide no college credit hours in any health curricula.

What I have is a PhD in marketing with minors in economics and industrial relations (management) and a base of a bachelor and master of business administration. I have professor emeritus status and academic administrative experience. I have many certifications in a wide variety of esoteric subjects. I also have experience as a management consultant to numerous businesses of all sizes, including hospitals and health-care not-for-profits. And since 2008, I have been an eleventh-hour hospice volunteer.

Fearful of health-related accrediting agencies, a university vice president to whom my dean friend reported said no to the proposed online NDE course. Half-jokingly, she said to me, "If we could just make it about managing."

"Great idea," I replied.

Lots more restructuring and research later, I submitted a new syllabus under a more expansive umbrella. The NDE would be used along the path to understanding broad, applied management concepts in a health-care environment. My credentials would survive accrediting scrutiny. Unfortunately, the subject itself would not survive university vice-presidential fears: loosely stated, "But she might say something about talking to dead people."

Certainly that would be true, but I do not want to get ahead of myself. The results of my research and my personal experiences will unfold in this book. Stories of patients, family members, and health-care professionals will transport us from mundane thinking to remarkable possibility. We will be bedside for unexpected visits and conversations with those no longer in physical bodies or with others perceived as angels. We will look at mistakes and at successes in journeying with our dying loved ones. We will examine ways to manage end-of-life experiences and learn how our communication styles may affect outcomes. We will share the exhilaration of knowing ways a deceased loved one is nearby. We will be reminded that such experiences are not new and that current technology reinforces our ways of knowing. Though I no longer feel the need to create a textbook to accompany an academic course, I do hope some may choose this book for that use. And as you read, there may be times you need to suspend your disbelief so that you are able to remain open to experiences and to needs of those nearing the end of life … that is, as some might say, of life in a physical body.

We'll look at the ways we involve ourselves in the end times of others. In her 1969 book, *On Death and Dying*, pioneer physician Elisabeth Kübler-Ross championed the seriously ill patient's right to express a treatment opinion and to participate in treatment. She argued for patient-inclusive decisions, for the patient's right to be heard, and for honoring the patient's feelings and wishes.[1] Along with respectful loved ones and professional caregivers, we will travel personally altering or unexpected journeys of sometimes intense, life-exit patient desires and experiences.

Because reading these real stories of real people allows us to listen—to hear them speak. We can think about ways, whether at hospital, home, or any other place, that we are a part of the final act of someone else's play while in an intermediary act of our own. Together, we can enjoy a love-filled and life-enhancing journey. Perhaps you'll also examine yourself, your patients, and your loved ones in ways that help you appreciate personal stories that are known and those not yet told—those you may discover. We can use this opportunity to explore possibilities that surround but are sometimes denied or denigrated by traditional thinking. And if you will, we can have loving fun together.

1

The Impossible as Possible

When I started writing this book, I had no idea that during this time, I would experience the ends of the lives of five close friends, two family members, and a beloved Scottish terrier. One friend was Bev. Though she is no longer here in a physical body, she continues to be my friend. And as you will read, her story is remarkable.

Life approaching its end, whether for someone younger when it is surprising or for someone older when death is more expected, can be something like a symphony's final movement. It may cleanse emotions or cause despair. It may lessen the tensions built over a lifetime. It may lift you up. It can be beautiful, but it isn't always. Parts of Bev's ending symphony, and that of her husband's, inform us of wondrous possibilities. Their remarkable end-of-life experiences are explorations into the impossibly possible.

I ask you, in reading Bev's story and additional later stories, to suspend your disbelief. Especially to those of you who want to demand absolute, scientific proof, I ask you to read and withhold judgment. I ask you to suspend disbelief, because loving to the end … and on can take us to unexpected places.

The first time I heard Bev's voice, she was crying. Bev and I began our lifelong friendship in the nursery of the hospital where we were born two days apart. Always close, she'll help us begin our exploration, introducing ideas and actualities expanded in later chapters. Bev's story includes examples of deathbed visions, multidimensional communications, shared death experiences, and after-death communications, along with other aspects of end-of-life caring. Together, we hope you'll remain open to possibility—to adventure into the end … and on.

After divorcing her college sweetheart and father of her three children, Bev had met an older man, Reggie, who became the love of her life. Many years of marriage later, Reggie had a series of small strokes over several years that resulted in his lessening ability to be fully present as he slowly became unable to care for himself. A larger stroke in his eighty-fifth year left him increasingly nonresponsive; he was dying, very slowly.

As a retired medical technician, Bev took specifics of care and decline in stride, but she struggled with the emotional stress of losing her love. And she wondered why he could not let go.

On a Sunday morning in October 2012, I felt a strong need to be with her. Sometime previously, I had taken the Hemi-Sync recording series *Going Home* to Bev so that she could listen to those recordings designed to help the family and so that Reggie could listen to those recordings designed to assist him in dying—in leaving his physical body. Neither had ever embraced my comfort with expanded life possibilities, but Bev figured they had nothing to lose.

I drove to her home and was greeted at the door by her eldest child, who had driven more than 250 miles with her own daughter, both of them nurses, to be there. Reggie's pulse and heartbeat were weakening, his body temperature was dropping, and mottling had begun in his extremities. He was actively dying, but very, very slowly. The slowness was taking its toll. Never had I seen my friend Bev look so sad—never.

I sat at the breakfast room table with Bev, her daughter, and her granddaughter, and I tried to sense Reggie. As someone who, for most of my life, has been connected in various ways to those no longer in physical bodies, I had become a hospice volunteer, and I was accustomed to the emotions of families who have a dying loved one. I hoped to sense the reason Reggie just kept struggling and hanging on. My friend's sad face and body posture were too much; it hurt to see her that way.

Finally, I asked whether she minded if I went to Reggie's room to be with him for a few minutes. She dispassionately mumbled, "Sure, go back there if you want."

A private home-health-care nurse was in the room, about to leave. We discussed some of the physical end signs and sounds that Reggie was presenting. Still, he was hanging on.

Shifting my mental awareness, I greeted Reggie and was answered with his radiant smile—not on his physical face, but through some mysterious, nonphysical communication pathway. So, staying in that pathway, I shared with him our wondering at his physical tenacity. His response: "I have some tidying up to do."

My return query: "What kind of tidying up?"

He simply repeated, "I have some tidying up to do."

This exchange was not spoken; no words were vocally expressed. I physically grinned. He grinned in that nonphysical space where we were communicating. I left the room and returned to where the others were sitting.

"Bev," I said, "Reggie just gave me a big smile and told me that he's still here because he has some tidying up to do." She sat there, still dejected, nodding her head at my disclosure and putting up with her friend's claims and beliefs. But then she jerked her head up and asked, "What did you say he said?"

"I told you he said he has some tidying up to do. I have no clue what that means. Tidying up?"

"Lynn, he used to say that all the time. That was a phrase he used all the time."

But I had never heard him use it.

And with that, she was smiling—her big, warm, usual smile. With the use of that "tidying up" phrase, she decided that I truly had made contact, somehow, some way. Then she wanted to hear again about the smile I had perceived, his seeming to be fine, and a few other details.

The home-health-care nurse had left. Bev's daughter and granddaughter remarked that they were hungry, and they asked whether I could stay with Bev so they could get takeout from a favorite seafood restaurant to bring back.

"Of course," I replied.

After they left, Bev was more animated. We got up from the table and walked into a room closer to Reggie's room. While we were standing there talking, Reggie came in, visible to me in that nonphysical, consciousness space we could access together. He was dressed in a sailor uniform and doing a silly dance, his big grin getting even bigger. I was having a hard time both paying attention to Bev and watching Reggie. Finally, I said, "Bev, I have to ask, did Reggie ever wear some navy uniform and dance around?"

"Why?"

"Because he's doing that right here, right now."

She laughed. He was in the navy as a very young man, which if I knew, I had forgotten. But, for sure, I had not known that every year, for years, to prove he could still fit in it, he would put on his uniform at Christmas and do a silly dance throughout the house. Later, Bev looked for some of the pictures to show to me and to others to whom she later told the story.

The girls came back with the food. Bev excitedly told them about the uniform and the dancing.

I did not go home immediately, but I visited another friend that afternoon. I had left my cell phone turned off during the afternoon.

A couple of hours later, I returned home. Though unusual for me, I immediately checked the home landline phone for messages. The first one was from Bev's daughter, who said, "Lynn, Reggie died about twenty minutes after you left." The second message was from Bev, who laughingly said in an uplifted, teasing voice, "Lynn, you killed my husband. Call me." The third message was again from her daughter, who told me how she, her daughter, and Bev had all three been in the room with Reggie when he took his last breath. Even more thrilling to them than being there in that moment was their experience with him. They wanted me to hear the whole story.

Gathered around his bed, holding his hand, or touching his arm, looking lovingly at him, Bev thought she needed to be saying a prayer, and she was trying to remember words when she realized her daughter was already reciting the twenty-third Psalm.

Her daughter asked whether Bev would like to listen to Reggie's heart as it was slowing, very gradually ceasing to beat. With trepidation, she agreed and put her head to his chest. With his heart's last beat, Reggie left, briefly taking Bev with him. She was exuberant when she told me about the experience of their consciousnesses departing their bodies together, its beauty, and, most of all, its intimacy, which she said exceeded any and all of their considerable physical intimacy in their twenty-nine years and ten months of a very happy marriage.

Graciously, she gave me credit for opening the way for that to happen—kind, but maybe not accurate. I remember Reggie telling me he had some tidying up to do. I think, maybe, my sensing the need to be with Bev that morning had been instigated by Reggie. But he had more to do. Within minutes after Reggie's last breath, Bev turned in the doorway to his room to see their Presbyterian minister standing there. He told her that, as soon as services were over, he felt like he needed to be there with them and had driven directly from church. Twenty minutes later, a close friend in another city called Bev, one who had not done so in about six months, but who said she just felt like she needed to call. "Tidying up," indeed.

Because this happened about fifteen months before I wrote their story, I asked Bev to take a look at what I had written for verification or for changes she felt needed to be made. She said what few inaccuracies there might be would be too minuscule to matter, as they wouldn't change the gist of the story at all. "And," she added, "funny you should be thinking about this now. I went to a noonday communion service at our church today, and we sang 'The Lord Is My Shepherd,' and I had a vivid recollection of the day that Reggie died in my arms because I was saying the twenty-third Psalm when he took his last breath. I can never think of this Psalm without thinking of his gift to me when he died. It was the most wonderful thing I have ever experienced, and I will be ever thankful for that—and for you too—being there with me. I don't mind at all if you publish this story. It is a story worth being told."

And again, days later in church, Bev reexperienced the exalting intimacy of her sharing with Reggie the experience of his transition. She told me that because of their shared death experience, it had been the most wonderful day of her life and that her thoughts about death and dying were changed.

Months went by without a repetition of this experience, though with a continuing appreciation for it. Then, in early November 2014, we learned that Bev had been diagnosed with an abdominal sarcoma, a rare cancer. Though she had felt tired on occasion, she had not experienced alarming symptoms of any kind until traveling in Europe with a friend. She realized that she was tiring more easily and completely than was at all her norm. When she returned home, she made an appointment with her primary physician that led to other appointments.

The local oncologist ruled out surgery because of the size and nature of Bev's very vascular tumor. The doctor prescribed a drug, hoping to shrink it. Bev's condition was such that she had to begin with a partial dosage, increasing the amount slowly. The pain continued to increase, with prescribed drugs given for that. Bev resisted being drugged as much as she possibly could. Her children, who lived in other cities, followed their mother's wishes and made arrangements for in-home caregivers, augmented with care from Bev's many friends, to assist in keeping Bev in her own home.

She went to visit her daughters for Thanksgiving. They observed her increased weakness. After that visit, they alternated coming to her home to be with her. Her son, who lived in a neighboring state, came to live with and care for her for a few days. Though Bev's friends commented about the rapidity of her decline, until Christmas, Bev's children seemed to be in denial. Her diagnosis was but two months old.

By Christmas, her daughters had taken her for a second opinion to a specialist in the larger city where they both lived. The tumor had doubled in size; surgery was not possible. Her friends had been dubious about Bev's being able to make the trip; she did successfully. However, less than a month later, Bev was released from what had been excruciating pain of the cancer her older daughter had said "is sucking the life out of her." It had.

Like her beloved Reggie, did Bev provide glimpses of living beyond the body? Glimpses of "to the end … and on"? Yes. Bev's dad provided me with some during the final week of Bev's life.

During those last days of her life, both of Bev's daughters were with her in her home, as were residential nurses and hospice nurses. Getting enough control over the pain had proven difficult. There were nights Bev's daughters were awakened every few hours when she would call out, sometimes scream, "Mom, Dad, come here; come help me." They told me that they believed their mom was seeing her parents, an occurrence that has been documented in many cross-century accounts of deathbed visions.

On one of those nights, in my own home, I experienced a lucid dream, seeing myself walking up to a door. I opened the door and looked in the room, and a man, seated to my right just inside that door, turned around and looked at me. It was as if he were watching, guarding what was in the room. I saw no farther than the man; he was dressed in black slacks, a black jacket, and a small black hat. The hat was not a fedora type, not a cowboy type, not a baseball cap; it was small, and I could not quite figure it out. He turned his head around, looking at me over his left shoulder. It was Jim, Bev's deceased father! I was quite surprised. He had been a very quiet man, occasionally flashing a large grin, especially where his daughter was concerned. In fact, I was so surprised to see him that I forced myself to awaken, look at a clock, and note the time—four o'clock in the morning—while instructing myself to remember the time and the visit when I awakened in the morning, which I did.

It was several days before Bev's daughters told me about the nights of calling out. And then I shared my dream of their grandfather. When I was describing the hat that I could not categorize with certainty, the younger daughter said, "Oh, Lynn, that was the cap he wore when he was riding his bike. Don't you remember?" Well, no, I did not remember that hat, but I did remember his bicycle riding until late in a very long life into his nineties. In telling them the story, I recalled that I had felt confused that he did not speak to me, just sat quietly. On reflection, however, I laughed, saying that, if he had been talkative, I might have wondered about an impostor posing as Bev's father. My dream occurred during one of those painful nights the daughters listened to their mom calling for her mom and dad. Had he wanted me to tell her? The family? Had he wanted me to know, to be comforted that he was there?

Bev's life force weakened dramatically and quickly. On the morning of her death, I had felt the need to go to her house and be with her younger daughter, share some hugs, and see my friend who, by then, was clearly dying. I did not know that her older daughter had decided to stay. As a nurse, she could see that her mom's life force was slipping away. We shared stories and looked at family pictures, and I left around eleven to have lunch with childhood friends. Ordinarily, Bev would have been with us.

The daughters, a hospice nurse, and the critical care nurse

conferred and thought Bev had another day or two of slowly leaving her body. The younger daughter decided to drive the almost five hours home to be with her family, collect some clothes, and return in the morning. She had been gone just a couple of hours when Bev's vital signs showed marked deterioration.

Around three o'clock in the afternoon, my cell phone rang. It was Bev's older daughter apprising me of the situation. Until she told me, I did not know her sister had left a little after noon. I asked if she wanted me to come back; I told her I'd be there. This was Bev's daughter who had been with her at Reggie's bedside as he took Bev briefly with him on the journey out of his body … and on.

I was offered the gift of love, of trust, and of spiritual opportunity. I called my husband and told him I might not see him at all that night. When I arrived at Bev's house, I learned the younger sister was on the road, en route home. The older sister and I hugged for a long time. Then we went to check on Bev. End-of-life signs were clearly accelerating. We hugged some more and hugged the experienced sitter who was attending to whatever needs might arise. Loving is so very important.

As we walked away from the room, we discussed whether big sis should call little sis to tell her that the remaining time was going to be much shorter. It was her decision to let her sister know but with no clarity on coming back that night or in the morning.

We heard a call from the sitter in Bev's room, telling us to come back. The signs were clear. Just as the cancer itself had grown so fast, so was Bev's journey from her body now moving rapidly. I was able to hold her hand and stroke the hair from her forehead as she was taking her last breaths. Her older daughter, with such love, said, "Mom, I'm going to say the twenty-third Psalm for you as we did for Reggie." With her head on her mom's chest, listening to her last breaths, she said the prayer, and she did so with such beauty, such love.

And I was getting a full-blown image of my lifelong friend with a big smile on her face. She was looking at us and looked beautiful, healthy, and happy—even with a bit of a quirky upturned lip, as though she was teasing me, "Doing your thing again?" As my thoughts turned to her daughter, the vision of Bev returned with a more serious expression, one that showed concern for her daughter's emotional well-being. I selfishly shifted energy and changed channels back to the smiling friend.

Tears, hugs, more tears, and more hugs. Deep breaths. And then it was time to make the first of many phone calls to be made. Hospice help arrived; the things that needed to be done began to be done. I was home that night by seven, leaving the older sister with one of her closest childhood friends, who came immediately after she was called.

Bev had made the decision for her younger daughter. She would not return that night; Bev was not there. A few days later, when I was visiting with that daughter, I told her of the visions at Bev's bedside. Her chatty daughter responded with more stories, hardly stopping to breathe. While she was talking, I began hearing another voice in a different space of knowing. It sounded and felt like Bev, but the two simultaneous conversations were competing, making neither fully coherent for me.

Tears welling up, I interrupted the daughter, "Hush, let's be quiet a minute. I'm hearing something from your mom."

In the quiet, Bev told me "I am so proud of my girls." Though I cannot precisely describe the context of what I heard, it was clear she was commenting on what they had been able to do to take care of her in those two months of rapidly escalating crises of care.

As the tears flowed, I asked her daughter to stand up so we could hug. We hugged and cried and cried and hugged. I could still feel Bev's presence and the love she was sending. I hoped her daughter could feel it too, so I asked her to clear her head of thought and place her attention in her chest, in the region of her heart. I opened my heart area in hopes that as we hugged, together we would feel the love from her mom. In similar circumstances, even with people I had not previously known, I had been able to share love across dimensions. Was this time a success? We think, yes, a little.

Like so many families, Bev's was with her, loving to the end ... and on. They could entertain the possibility of survival beyond physical life. Some cannot but can talk of loved ones living on in memories or in serendipitous events, as will be explored in a later chapter.

In little ways throughout our lives, each of us has been preparing for end-of-life love. Do you remember childhood playtimes when someone got hurt? A friend was bruised or bleeding? Or you were? Do you remember how much it helped to have someone there with you, maybe just there waiting with you, waiting for an adult, maybe, who knew what to do and the best way to get you to safety?

You were learning, then, the power of staying to the end ... and on. That was early life practice in learning ways to support and love in good times, not so good times, and really tough times, until you were either beyond the crisis or you had learned to live with changes you would rather have not happened and to keep on living and loving, no matter what.

From childhood, then, you've rehearsed end-of-life care, except that it wasn't quite the same. In today's modern health-care world, there can be large numbers of caregivers, some very specialized. And the people involved can be continuously changing. The exploration in this book is about traversing the shifting demands of loving as end of life approaches, completes, and often leads on.

If you are a family member, you have needs and responsibilities that are personal, often heartrending. If you are a professional caregiver, you have career requirements and expectations, but you are also a human who has your own heart stuff. Together, you are the music and the musicians of a symphony, a piece of music played by a combination of instruments. You are life's caregiving music and its players, learning as you go, creating a symphony of love.

2

Decisions Best Guided by Love

The stories of Reggie and Bev are windows for observing physical life endings. Reggie was in his eighties and had a series of strokes, leading to his slow demise. Bev was in her seventies and experienced an unexpected diagnosis, followed by a rapid disease progression. I remember, a week or so before her death, standing by her bed, observing her writhing in the pain they had yet to get under control. She reached her hand out to mine, and I held it gently, holding back my tears when she said, "I don't want to live like this."

Those and other situations ultimately confront each of us. We have decisions to make, often complicated. We have to work with others. Even then, the outcomes of our family or professional decisions may not end as we would like; it helps to remember to be guided by love. Death may be approaching, unexpected and in camouflage. Another story, one of my own, is illustrative.

There, in front of me, is this really old, shriveled, bent man in a wheelchair with blood splattered on his matching robe and pajamas, three hundred thread-count blue cotton, piped in navy. The blood must be fresh, because it's red, not that dried rusty-brown, and there's lots of it.

I stand there, looking at this in horror and wondering who slipped me some mind-bending something. Remembering I haven't had anything to eat or drink in about six hours, I conclude this aberration must be real. A fuzzy voice, my own, asks where the bloodied, wheeled wonder can get something to drink, because he's had nothing pass his lips in hours. An officious woman responds that it's self-service, that way, pointing around a corner and down a hall. *Is she nuts?* I'm thinking, but I look in the direction she points.

Immediately, in my head, I'm singing, "I'm trippin', oh, yes, indeed, I'm trippin'." Damn. Jerry Lee Lewis pounding on my inner keyboard and bellowing out "I'm trippin'." What else can it be? Down that hall? There, lying strapped to a rolling bed, is a naked chest with a head hanging down almost to the floor, it's mouth screaming, "Where's my wife? Tell that bitch to git herself back here now! Goddam, git back here, woman."

I want out of there fast. Forcing myself to focus, I look at the bloodied, wheelchaired, ninety-eight-year-old man in front of me with renewed concern for him—he's my father. My sister is standing there, eyes wide with freckles and age spots all faded from view. What have we done? Is there a way out?

I hear my sister's voice. "When can his attendants, his caregivers, come here to stay with him? Can I call them now, from here? He has to have help with almost everything."

The people on the other side of the desk are looking at her, at the three of us, as though we are the most inept and ignorant people possible. Looking back, we just may have been.

We were at the admissions desk of the psychiatric unit in a hospital. How did we get there? We got there in a manner that normally we never would have allowed.

Though Mom had died eighteen years previously, Dad had continued to live alone in their home. With the onset of macular degeneration in his eighties, he began to need assistance. When he was about ninety (exact timing escapes me now), he had a brief hospitalization and returned home in a more weakened state, which necessitated round-the-clock care. We were fortunate to find help for him, although his increased dependency, coupled with the changing physiology and neurology of his aging mind and body, was very difficult for him—for all of us. His long-time primary care physician suggested he see a specialist.

For a couple of years, that was a good thing. Dad even wrote a family history. He continued to get a variety of prescriptions for medication from several physicians. I remember his occasional strange, brief outbursts—totally beyond our ability to manage. During good days, which was most of the time, he would tell us how much he appreciated what we were doing and that he knew how difficult it could be … reminding us also of how many older family members had been his responsibility. When we asked the doctors questions, they were only partially answered, if at all. Some physicians wanted to call in another prescription and still another one. We were unclear about interactions among the drugs and concerned about changes, given Dad's age. My brother, sister, and I were heartsick and lost. And that is the how and the why my master-degree-from-Bryn-Mawr sister and my PhD-self were standing like fools behind locked doors at a psychiatric ward desk with our wheelchair-bound father.

That doesn't explain the blood on my father. A specialist had told us he would regulate the medications, but only in the psychiatric ward of a specified hospital. We were to take him to its emergency room for evaluation and admitting, and he would call ahead to tell them we were coming. We went; we waited hours. Dad's body was without food, water, and his scheduled medications—not a good way to keep him balanced. Finally, we were taken to an examination area, and a charming young physician came in. His first question to Dad was not met with a pleasant response. And as simple, basic questions were asked, Dad became increasingly agitated with the seeming insult of such inanity. Even sick and old, Dad was not stupid. I suppressed a smile when, somewhere in the process, Dad showed his displeasure with the endurance game he felt he was being forced to play. He was more than ready to go home and said so. We wanted to take him out of there.

Our choice for straightening out his medications had been limited to this single one by his physicians. When the admission process had been completed, a large, strong orderly was sent in to take us to the psychiatric unit to admit Dad there. By then, Dad had decided if what had been done was the best the hospital could offer, he wanted none of it. I couldn't blame him for thinking that way. My heart hurt for him and for us. We were bereft but soldiered on, sticking to the plan for a longer-term benefit.

Dad decided to fight the orderly and to resist being wheeled anywhere. The strength of his college boxing, adult tennis, and golf playing returned as he grabbed the doorsill to resist transport. The orderly overwhelmed his ninety-eight-year-old wheelchair captive to strap him down. Thin and increasingly aged skin tore in several places. There was a lot of blood. Ironically, Dad had become the enemy and the victim of the caregivers who were trying to help him. My sister and I had become collateral damage, sheep still following medical orders, leading our father and ourselves to his psychiatric pen.

Dad was placed in a single room within sight of the nurses' desk. We stayed with him, making sure his wounds were treated before we were told to leave.

The next day we were outside the ward awaiting entry during designated visiting hours. There were three times: one in the morning, one at noon, and another in early evening. For a couple of days, at least two of the three of us siblings were there at each visiting time. We would have continued that but were informed by a nurse that only one at a time could visit. Then we were told none of us could be there at noon, which was the physician's time for making rounds. It is an understatement to say that we were alarmed at how easily a single physician could unilaterally dismiss Dad's family care unit.

But what about Dad? Just a few highlights. He was forced to spend time in the ward's group room "to learn to socialize." At the time of his hospitalization, Dad had one remaining living friend who, at ninety-eight, was also restricted in his physical capacity; they talked often on the phone. At home, Dad had been visited daily by some of his children, grandchildren, or great-grandchildren. He had been visited frequently, also, by our friends, who loved him like a father. He knew how to socialize. What he did not know was how to fraternize with a half-naked, strapped-to-a-gurney man screaming obscenities at his wife. That seemed absurd—still does. Is there any reason an accomplished, long-lived, well-mannered man, one who had served on numerous boards of directors, which included that of a hospital, needs to learn psychiatric-ward-blessed social skills? Is there any reason the family needed to consent to what felt increasingly like elder abuse? Was this for the convenience of an attending physician or for the benefit of the patient? Was there no more loving way to accomplish what was needed?

Was there some reason Dad had to live with other ward residents walking in and out of his room, getting in and out of his bed? Was there some reason he was expected to eat foods he had not chosen to eat in years or, alternatively, have nothing to eat at all?

If Dad wanted water, he was told he had to walk to the social room and get it. He could not have it in his room. Our bloodied, sight-restricted hero was told to get up, find his walker, and walk down the hall to get some water … and to make this work while his age-weakened body was adjusting to dramatic changes in medications.

It's not hard to understand that Dad became both thinner and weaker. Yes, his occasional outbursts stopped. His medications were changed; I can't remember if there were fewer of them. He was calmer. Before we could take him home, I had to meet with each of his at-home caregivers. We had continued to pay them for the weeks he was hospitalized so that they would not seek nor accept other jobs. I had to tell each of them that a different man was coming home, a man in need of much more care. Several quit, feeling unprepared for the elevated level of care. We found others who were angels on earth.

The dad we had taken to the hospital never returned. Eventually, we sought help from hospice. There was no specific disease. He did not meet hospice criteria until I remembered that he had a brief period of home-health care during a short illness about six months prior. Thankfully, I had kept those records. His weight was significantly lower; that last finding, added to other itemized factors, was enough to qualify him for hospice.

And what a blessing to have qualified for hospice! Kind, considerate, trained workers checked on him and on us regularly. They evaluated and reevaluated his need for medications that kept him calm and eased whatever pain he encountered in the process of his body's shutting down. They made certain we knew what to do, how to do it, and when to call them for additional help. And they tutored us in knowing what to observe so that when the active dying process began, we would call them. They assured us they would also take care of having a death certificate legally signed, and they would call for our chosen funeral provider to come for his body. They would take care of business and give us the space to love.

Six months after our dad entered the hospital for medication modification, he died at home, the place he had wanted to be. His death certificate read: "Cause of death: failure to thrive."

And yes, there was love, a lot of it. Still is.

In the years since, what I did not know then, what I did not recognize has become more apparent. We will walk together through some of that in a later chapter. And I am sure we will learn more as we go, delving into experiences during end of life, remembering to suspend disbelief. The possibilities are amazing, often exhilarating.

3

Resuscitated Life

Not everyone lives to be in their seventies, eighties, or nineties. Not everyone has a serious disease. Some have accidents. Some die for unknown reasons.

And some technically die but are resuscitated. Many do not report experiences of sensing they have died and come back, but many do. They have had what is now being called a near-death experience (NDE). Previously, and in other cultures, you might hear about imminent death or the border of death or provisional death or almost death. Some physicians have argued strongly that anyone whose heart has stopped is dead, and they argue against any modifying terms. People who return from states of clinical death are said to do so only because someone has found a way to resuscitate them; otherwise, their death would not have been reversed. Such events, however, are not new.

While reading a book he discovered in an antique shop in France, a physician and archeologist named Dr. Philippe Charlier found a description of a patient who had been a famous pharmacist in Paris. The patient was temporarily unconscious and then reported seeing a light of such purity and brightness he suspected he had been in heaven. That book, *Anecdotes de Médecine,* was written by Pierre-Jean du Monchaux (1733–1766), a military physician from northern France, and contains what may be among the oldest discovered medical reports of a near-death experience.[2] Dr. Charlier has compared the almost 250-year-old description with current NDE criteria developed in the 1980s by Dr. Bruce Greyson and has published those affirming results in the journal *Resuscitation.*[3]

In 1975 in his book *Life After Life,* Dr. Raymond Moody created the term *near-death experience* (NDE). Since then, there has been an explosion of research, internet first-person accounts, books, and movies that reveal and explore the possible meanings of such events. Prior to discussions of NDEs, there was something called the Lazarus phenomenon. It has been described as occurring in patients who had been clinically dead and then either resuscitated or had a spontaneous circulatory return. With suppressed brain activity, those patients might describe a subjective experience, visitors, and other events. And, in addition to symptoms such as anxiety, depression, insomnia, and nightmares, patients also reported sensory phenomena such as moving through a tunnel, seeing a light, or feelings of having left the body. These events had been given insufficient attention. Dr. Moody's research changed that.

As I personally learned more and more about NDEs and their impact on the experiencer and their families, I decided to reach out to share what I had learned. I offered a continuing education course at a nearby university: The Healing Gifts of Near-Death Experience (NDE), Nearing Death Awareness (NDA), and After-Death Communication (ADC). Its description read as follows: "Popular movies and TV shows depict NDEs, NDAs, and ADCs, often without fully portraying a sense of just how healing each can be for the experiencer and all those around him/her, including family, friends, caregivers. The printed media increasingly give recognition to the abundance of serious research into these aspects of living. For instance, the Wall Street Journal on August 3, 2006 (D1) included an article, 'For Many Bereaved Families, "Visits" From Late Loved Ones Provide Solace.' In this seminar, we'll explore NDEs, NDAs, and ADCs, and we'll learn more about how the dying communicate with us, may continue to do so after death, and how healing often results. You are encouraged to come with your own stories and questions." The course objectives included introducing participants to the research studies of NDEs, NDAs, and ADCs; validating the experiences of participants and their families; and providing a venue for discussions, including the science behind the phenomena, experiential reporting, and explorative dialogue.

Enrollment for that course was double the expectation. That was the catapult for creating an affiliate group of the International Association for Near-Death Studies (IANDS). People needed a venue for discussion and validation, and I thought having a free, easily available one to be a worthy goal. A local library agreed to provide space for a monthly meeting at a branch location. Though it has never grown large, the group continues to meet.

Sometimes an experiencer comes, tells his whole story, gets hoped-for acceptance and reinforcement, and never comes again. Some come regularly for a few years, some for longer. One man in his early fifties came to share the NDE he had at the age of five. He had internalized it, like a cyst just beneath the surface, never sharing it with his family, fearing scorn or derision. The meeting allowed him to lance that cyst, to be appreciated, and to be believed. He came to one more meeting before he was diagnosed with a life-ending disease. A woman in her late thirties attended for several years. As a cradle-Episcopalian, she felt she could not share it with other church members; her husband did not want to talk about it. When she was well enough to go back to work, she got a job as a funeral cosmetologist—a quite comfortable environment for her. Having no one locally available, experiencers have driven four hours or more from towns in neighboring states, eager to tell their stories and to have their experiences acknowledged. One local woman who carried a written account of her NDE in her purse found out about our local meeting and noted its time and place on her written account; two years later, she finally came, read the account to us, and was supported and encouraged. Though we never saw her again, we remember her still.

Definitions and descriptions of a near-death experience may differ slightly; most will include some spiritual, transcendental, or otherworldly occurrence that may happen during a close or possibly imminent death or dying incident. The IANDS website describes an NDE as a distinctly subjective experience. And the website explains that a person may be clinically dead or near death and that, additionally, there are people who, in deep meditation, profound grief, or a momentary shift in consciousness, have reported similar experiences.

Many reports include similarities. Often included are viewing your own body from outside the body, hearing conversations nearby or in other locations while not conscious, locating yourself at a place distant from the actual location of your body, seeing other living persons not in the proximity of your body, seeing known deceased persons, experiencing a sense of peace, seeing a powerful and beautiful light, being embraced by feelings of profound love, and/or experiencing a review of your life.

As a teenager, retired FBI agent Vanessa was exhausted from being pounded by strong ocean waves when she experienced a different kind of consciousness. Having sailed with her parents to a small island in the Gulf of Mexico, just off of Dauphin Island, Alabama, she and her boyfriend had walked around to the south side of the island where they ventured into the surf. Unexpectedly, they realized the waves and their undertow were stronger than expected. As Vanessa fought the surf's brutal strength, she knew she could not make it. As she relaxed into that feeling, she remembers feeling as though she was enveloped in beautiful white light, and she felt very peaceful even though she knew she was drowning. Her larger, stronger boyfriend had other ideas and somehow managed to get them both onto the shore. Decades later, Vanessa told me about her similar-to-NDE episode and relived its beauty and calmness. "That is what I would like to tell people who have had a loved one drown. I had always thought drowning would be a horrible experience; it wasn't. The beauty and peace have stayed with me; I do not fear death."

Dr. Mary Neal is a board-certified orthopedic spine surgeon who drowned in 1999 while kayaking on a Chilean river. In her book, *To Heaven and Back: A Doctor's Extraordinary Account of Her Death, Heaven, Angels, and Life Again: A True Story* (2011), she describes her NDE and tells of going to heaven and back, conversing with Jesus, and experiencing God's enveloping love. Dr. Neal admits she had a fear of possible horrors of drowning, and while drowning, was acutely aware of everything that was happening. She describes her experience as being contrary to the horrors she had feared.[4]

Perhaps surprisingly, the IANDS website reports that

approximately 10 percent of patients who experience cardiac arrest in hospital settings report an NDE. Many near-death experiencers (NDErs) feel the term *near-death* is incorrect. They suggest *in-death* is more accurate than *near-death* and also caution that actively integrating the personal changes resulting from an NDE often takes years.

The most thorough source for NDE information is available from IANDS, founded in 1978.[5] There is a related group with overlap in interest and research, the American Center for the Integration of Spiritually Transformative Experiences (ACISTE).[6] ACISTE supports people who have had spiritually transformative experiences (STEs), i.e., a profound life-changing spiritual experience, one that may take months or years to integrate into their lives.

Even with massive numbers of first-person interviews, research studies, and conferences focused on NDEs in the forty-plus years since the term NDE was coined, there are those who choose to ignore, denigrate, or deny even their possibility. There are others, however, who continue to explore what, if, and in what ways, might such an event occur and what it might teach us about life and death. In knowing those things, might we not be helped in caring for dying loved ones?

For our purposes, finding the love messages is really important. I am not an NDEr, but I have had related things happen throughout my life. For that reason, I embrace the importance of providing support, of accepting and applauding the possibilities NDErs report. More and more, medical teams are also providing corroboration of NDErs' stories.

Writing for Salon.com, and adapted from his book, *Brain Wars,* Mario Beauregard, associate research professor at the Departments of Psychology and Radiology and the Neuroscience Research Center at the University of Montreal, describes, in gripping detail, brain surgery that required singer/songwriter Pam Reynolds to agree to a surgery nicknamed "Operation Standstill," an extreme procedure necessitating that she essentially die so that she could possibly live.[7] During surgery when she was clinically dead, Pam experienced elements commonly described in near-death and out-of-body experiences. Even though her eyes had been taped shut and molded earpieces eliminating external sounds had been taped in, she later was able to tell the surgical team specific things she had heard and observed during surgery. They verified her observations.

In his 1994 book, *Parting Visions,* Dr. Melvin Morse provides wonderful stories of possibility. In one he recounts the story of a rancher who accurately described his unusual resuscitation to one of the attending nurses when she visited his room the next day.

Dr. Morse also recalls reports from clinically dead children he has resuscitated. He describes ways children repeatedly have given precise details of their own resuscitations. For instance, one told about seeing the doctor put a tube in his nose. And another told about seeing his doctor use paddles on him that "sucked" him back into his body.[8]

Many NDErs tell stories of visiting loved ones in "heaven," where they have beautiful, loving experiences. Not all visit. A friend recently told me of his experience, anesthetized, during surgery, of suddenly feeling as though he was in a dusky spiral being moved away from himself while hearing himself saying, "I don't want to go; I don't want to go," and then being out of the tunnel and back in his post-surgery body. Reported NDE experiencer numbers are massive and growing and are too numerous to ignore.

Some of us may want to say, "So what," or to counter with all sorts of possibilities. A more loving thing to do is to admit we have limited knowledge and information and to support each other – to be open, accepting, and encouraging. Dr. Michael Sabom, an Atlanta, Georgia, cardiologist who frequently performed cardiopulmonary resuscitations was a non-believer until he did a study in the emergency room, finding that, when interviewed sensitively and within a few days of successful resuscitation, 43% of people told him about NDEs.[9] In his book, *Light and Death,* Dr. Sabom suggests that simply reading stories of NDEs may not decrease skepticism. He challenges us to stand within four feet of experiencers, look into their eyes, and watch for their authentic tears. If you do that, he predicts skepticism will diminish and perhaps leave altogether.[10]

I agree with Dr. Sabom. The extraordinary stories told by ordinary individuals should challenge even the most hard-core skeptic. Certainly, all of us can agree that we have no absolute understanding of consciousness. There are those who maintain that without brain function, there is no consciousness, but even that is challenged by stories such as Mario Beauregard's regarding Pam Reynolds's experience.

When Dr. Eben Alexander, an academic neurosurgeon, wrote in *Proof of Heaven* (2012) of his own NDE during a deep coma brought on by a brain infection, there was an explosion of interest. Similarly, when nurse Penny Sartori, PhD, published her book, *Wisdom of Near-Death Experiences: How Understanding NDEs Can Help Us Live More Fully* (2014), there was another surge in interest in the first-person stories that were the heart and soul of the extensive research on which her book is based.

Internationally renowned cardiologist Dr. Pim von Lommel systematically researched NDEs. The stories his patients told him were difficult for him to accept, especially given his findings that during the NDE, an inverse relationship seems to appear between clarity of consciousness and loss of brain function. He also could not explain that people across cultures and ages report similar experiences. His 2011 book is based on his extensive research. *Consciousness Beyond Life, the Science of the Near-Death Experience* offers scientific evidence of the near-death phenomenon and of experiencing consciousness beyond the body.

Over a period of years, three-time NDEr, P.M.H. Atwater, LHD, PhD (Hon.), has written fifteen books and numerous articles on NDEs. Using police investigative methods of observation and interviewing that she learned from her police officer father, her research differs from more academic sources, with some clinically verified and included in the Dutch study published in Lancet, 2001. The evidence she presents is personal and poignant. On her website is a very helpful tool for experiencers, caregivers, and family members. It is the largest section devoted to aftereffects and how to handle those that exist; some information is repeated on the NDE aftereffects page at the IANDS website.[11]

At the Monroe Institute, Scott Taylor, EdD, is the facilitator of a program designed to help anyone release the fear around dying by simulating the near-death experience.[12] His own NDE was that of a 1981 shared death experience with a young boy, and it changed his life. He assists program participants in exploring the nonphysical universe and visiting the realms encountered by NDErs. Dr. Taylor also serves on the board of IANDS.

And during end-of-life care, you may also be helped at the IANDS website by reading "Near-Death Experiences and Nearing Death Awareness in the Terminally Ill," written by Pamela M. Kircher, MD; Maggie Callanan, RN, CRNH; and the IANDS board of directors. The descriptions of nearing death awareness as part of the dying process are especially poignant and helpful.[13] The authors encourage allowing your loved ones to talk about their awareness, because the last stage of life often provides the most powerful interactions that loved ones have had or will have in an entire lifetime.

Some of the interactions may lead to continuing communication without the existence of a living physical body. Some may open a pathway to expanded awareness and an openness to possibility.

4
Communicating Nonphysically

One night I was awakened by the presence of my friend, Brazilian shaman Ipu, who was also known as Dr. Bernardo Peixoto, a consultant to the Smithsonian Institute in Washington, DC. I couldn't see him; I didn't hear him say anything; I simply felt as though he was there in the room with me. I felt this so strongly that I looked at the clock and noted the time, which I think was two o'clock in the morning, but this was some years ago, and I am no longer certain. Around six o'clock that morning, when my husband and I began our day, I told him about feeling as though Ipu had been in our room earlier. Later that morning, when I went to my office, turned on my computer, and began reading my emails, I had one telling me that Ipu had died in Washington at the same time I had felt him in my room in Mobile, Alabama. I expect, with some certainty, many others received that inexplicable departure nod of friendship from Ipu.

A lot of years have gone by since I realized I could receive messages from people without the need for them to be in my presence or to have written me a letter or to have called me on the telephone or to have sent a text message or email or to even be alive. I delved into figuring out why and in what ways that could possibly happen. I'm still looking for those answers.

I have found none of us is alone. I have received many messages from people I knew and people I had not known during their stay here on Earth, in physical bodies. I still cannot explain it fully.

Ipu clearly was not physically in Mobile. His lifeless body was many miles away. So where was his consciousness? And if he could communicate after his physical death, might he have been able to do so before his physical birth? Some make clear cases for that very possibility. In *Life Between Life*, Dr. Joel Whitton and Joe Fisher tackle the questions of where do we come from, where do we go, and is there something like an in-between. They use modern techniques for unfolding the concepts across time and cultures referred to as bardo, gusho, Anjea, pardish, or metaconsciousness.[14] I've been told many stories, none of which I can fully explain.

Sarah spent Tuesdays with her brother, who had at-home hospice care. It was her day to be with him, freeing his wife to do some of those things that need to be done away from home. One Tuesday, as Sarah was leaving her home for her brother's house, she answered her phone. Hospice workers had called to tell her to hurry; her brother's illness had escalated, and death could be near. Driving there, Sarah recalls that she had the most peaceful feeling she has ever had, before or since. She looked at the car's clock. Later, she learned that feeling of indescribable peace occurred at her brother's time of death.

Is it really possible to be in touch with people at death or after? People who are no longer in their physical bodies? That depends on who you ask and what their belief systems might suggest. It also depends on what is meant by being in touch.

Perhaps you have been seeking a physical explanation. I am uncertain we will find one. We do research on the brain, thinking, as one friend of mine has said, "The world is too stuck with the notion that it has something to do with what's inside our skulls when we know that synapses firing are only correlates for physical expression and really don't control or have influence on thinking per se." We know that research of the brain has not explained mind or nonlocal reality or the soul. Even so, as we will see in a later chapter, we continue to use what we can, using metaphorical physiological linking of recorded brain frequencies to preferred thinking and communication styles. We lean on our local reality as a pathway to what may be beyond.

Few of us would disagree, however, that we stay in touch with those we love through memories, through shared events, and through the love stored deep inside. We look at pictures. We wear items of clothing or jewelry that make us feel close. We have celebrations. We say prayers and feel gratitude.

You may have read books, watched movies, seen newspaper articles, or done other things in an effort to know if you can really stay in touch with someone you love. Even unlikely sources, such as the *Wall Street Journal* on August 3, 2006 (section D1), have reinforced that possibility, publishing an article titled "For Many Bereaved Families, 'Visits' from Late Loved Ones Provide Solace."

Many of you who are reading this may have had interactive experiences or some kind of after-death communication. In fact, the concept of ghost stories has been societally pervasive for centuries. Unfortunately, many are disturbed, rather than delighted, by the possibility. Others have wonderfully gratifying experiences.

In the last years of my mom's life, she spent a lot of time sitting on a couch in the den. She admitted to me that she often felt the presence of a very loved, very intelligent, deceased wire-haired dachshund sitting by her feet, as though he was there to take care of her. She was comforted by his presence.

After pouring their hearts, souls, and physical energy into caring for loved ones until the last breath, some people begin to look for reminders or signs of reinforcement, such as birds, flowers, songs, or familiar smells. A friend told me that her mother had once pointed to a cardinal sitting in a backyard tree, saying one visited every year and sat in the same tree and that she looked forward to the cardinal's visit. Then, smiling, she casually and teasingly remarked, "If I ever come back to this earth, I think I'll come as a cardinal." After her mom died, the friend's sister was cleaning out their mom's house when she looked outside and saw not one, but a flock of cardinals in the tree, and it wasn't even the right season for them to be there. What to make of that? You decide. My friend took it as a message from her mom, allowing her to have loved to the end … and on.

Since her husband Warner's death, my friend Sandra and several family members have noticed a crow who appears when something personally meaningful is happening. The crow seems to make certain that he is noticed, which is the reason family members began asking each other about him. They believe it is a way that Warner has been able to get through to them.

Even though she was on vacation, Sarah felt a bit out of sorts. Near Yosemite, she and her husband were at a rest stop when she felt an urge to get out of their car and look up. She saw a dragonfly above her head and another farther up; then they were flying toward each other, touching and touching before flying off. She felt as though they were messengers of some kind. Because her mom had been ill, Sarah reached for her cell phone; it wouldn't work. In the meantime, her husband had gone into a nearby restroom where he was able to answer his phone's ring. When he returned to the car, he told Sarah that her mom had died. Reflecting later on the events of the day, Sarah realized that she had been watching the dragonflies at the exact time of her mother's death. She enjoys the possibility that, perhaps, she was seeing her mom being joyously greeted by her deceased father, touching and touching. With the giggle of her extraordinarily sunny sense of humor, Sarah told me that her mother hated bugs, so Sarah was all the more amused during her mother's funeral when she looked at the back wall of glass in the cemetery's chapel and saw a dragonfly. Just bugs, or representative visions of her mom? If you ask Sarah, as I did, she'll tell you it was her mom.

In 2006 a mother whose young son had died came to our local Mobile, Alabama, affiliate group of IANDS, not because either had near-death experiences, but because, soon after his death, he had begun "speaking" to her. She wanted to share her wonder and delight with others who would understand and appreciate her experiences. Using her son's messages as foundational material and since moving to the West Coast, that mother, Terri Daniel, has written several wonderful books, has become an ordained interfaith minister and grief counselor, and has created the annual Afterlife Awareness Conference, which features noted scientists, physicians, ministers, and mediums to help and comfort others in their quests for understanding a continuation of consciousness after death.[15]

In another dream experience of my own, I heard the deceased mother of a childhood friend asking me to call her son and tell him that he was not doing what she had repeatedly told him to do—to please tell him that. The next day I left a message on his answering machine at his home, several states and hundreds of miles away: "George, call me." When he returned my call, I repeated the message. Though he asked me several questions to possibly clarify the message, I could only tell him to try to remember what his momma had always wanted him to do. I ascertained, a few days later—and too late—that, quite possibly, his mom was urging him to have a physical checkup sooner than he had planned. Because of a business commitment, he had postponed his checkup by less than a week. Though he had looked and acted physically fit, he had a fatal heart attack two days prior to his postponed checkup. His father had also died abruptly, unexpectedly, from a heart attack. It made sense to me then, as it does now, that his mother would have wanted him to have regular physical examinations, with special attention to his heart's health. His wife told many of his business friends of the conversation we had, and at his funeral, they were anxious, curious, and some a bit reticent to meet the friend who had dreamed of George's mother with a premonitory warning.

Chiropractor, singer, and songwriter Annie Kagan was devastated by the accidental death of her older brother. Three weeks later she was startled by his voice awakening her. And his voice wasn't inside her head; it was outside. Dr. Kagan bravely tells her story in *The Afterlife of Billy Fingers, How My Bad-Boy Brother Proved to Me There's Life After Death*. In his introduction to the book, Dr. Raymond Moody says we, in Western civilization, falsely assume experiences like Annie Kagan's cannot be possible or that they might even be pathological.[16]

In the United States, for more than 135 years, those who believe in the continuity of life and the survival of personality beyond death, as well as those who are curious, have been able to visit, attend classes or services, or live on the grounds of the Lily Dale Assembly, a spiritualist community in New York State. A warm-climate alternative to Lily Dale, the fifteen-years-younger Cassadaga Spiritualist Camp is located near Daytona Beach, Florida. And in Essex, England, spiritualists from around the world attend Arthur Findlay College to study Spiritualist philosophy, religious practice, healing, spiritual, and related disciplines.[17] In each of these locations, individuals encounter the possibility or potentiality of being in touch with someone who is no longer in a physical body—someone who we would say has died.

Of course, you do not have to travel to have your own experience. Throughout my life, I have had many. For example, my deceased aunt awakened me one night, standing at the foot of my bed; my mother took me on an out-of-body flight into a most magnificent space, after which I returned to my body and realized tears were flowing down my face; my deceased friend Bev, who is featured earlier in this book, talked to me after her physical death and, during a phone call from her daughter who had called to tell me about her own daughter's engagement, even told me details of the bridal dress.

Communication with those no longer in physical bodies can happen in many ways. When I hear messages, it is usually in clairaudient form. When I see, it is clairvoyantly, or I feel clairsentiently, know through claircognizance, smell clairaliently, or use clairgustance for tasting.

We can use these same sensory possibilities in situations that do not involve communicating with those no longer in physical bodies. Michael Murphy and Rhea White, writing in *The Psychic Side of Sports*, give a variety of examples. For instance, they tell of two clairvoyant premonitory dreams, one in 1967 that influenced race car driver A.J. Foyt, allowing him to edge through a smash-up ahead of him and win his third Indianapolis 500. And they describe the dreaming of racehorse owner Ralph Lowe, in which his rider, the legendary Willie Shoemaker, would misjudge the finish of the 1957 Kentucky Derby, telling "the Shoe" about it the Friday night before the race, getting assurances that it would not happen, and then having it happen as dreamed.[18]

Scheduled to leave her home in Chicago for a lecture in Florida, while at O'Hare Airport, Dr. Elisabeth Kübler-Ross heard a voice (clairaudience) telling her not to board her scheduled flight. Knowing that a large audience would be waiting, she hesitantly boarded the plane and then heard the voice again. Reluctantly, she left the plane. It later crashed into the Everglades, killing everyone on board.[19]

Where do these premonitory dreams and voices come from? Where do the voices, smells, sights, thoughts, tastes, and knowings of our deceased loved ones come from? There are thousands of books, research studies, recorded lectures, websites, and movies that give possible answers. For our purposes, we care more about honoring the possibility in ways that allow us to love until the end ... and on.

I have been privileged to help friends do that. It is so important to be open and to simply report, rather than interpret. For instance, a pink rose to one person may be a love reminder, always received on Valentine's Day, while to another, it may mean sorrow, the flowers chosen for a loved one's funeral. Report, then, the pink rose you see, not associative information you might interpret. Simply allow your senses to inform you from a source that consciousness studies, brain scans, and the like may not yet explain. Inform and report, remembering that your personal bias may cause you to misinterpret the meaning of the information you have received.

A friend brought me a teddy bear given by her son Jim to his sister Hazel and asked me if I would mind sharing any information I might sense. The fact that Jim had died in an accident could have been information I picked up claircognizantly from my friend. What was more specific and helpful was picking up on Jim's laughter as he made fun of Hazel's toes and the way his sister danced or walked. When my friend told her daughter and one of her daughter's girlfriends those details, about which neither she nor I had known anything, they confirmed that Jim had teased Hazel about her toes, calling them little sausages and that he had always made fun of the way his sister danced. I knew neither of the girls; I only knew, postmortem, what Jim conveyed to me.

Another friend had come by my house to visit and talk about subjects of mutual interest. She is a professional woman, with several advanced degrees, who I have known for a few years. As I was enjoying an intellectual and esoteric discussion with her, I began to sense a presence standing behind her physical being. Knowing she would be amenable to my talking to her about a nonphysical presence, I tentatively mentioned something about perhaps sensing a son and asked her if she had a deceased son. She teared up, answering, "Yes."

Then I saw a series of images, one of which was a box beneath her bed, which I understood to be some of his things, so I described a few to her. Without going into great detail, the things I was able to describe confirmed to her that she had been contacted by her son who had died many years previously—a fact I had not known. Her tears of joy and gratitude were those of loving to the end ... and on—a gift she graciously shared with me.

A patient had been diagnosed with heart failure. One afternoon, his hospice nurse recognized decreasing responsiveness and other signs of physical deterioration. Later that evening, she noted that while in bed, he had picked up the remote for his television and held it to his ear, using it like a phone and talking for almost an hour to his deceased wife. As with other near-death patients, he said nothing that indicated any signs of confusion.[20]

I had not talked with or texted a good friend for several months when, on July 2, I suddenly felt the need to contact her. A few texts between us did not clarify why. No matter; it was good to be in touch. The next day, I again needed to contact her, giving recognition to the death of her adult son almost six months previously. As I texted, I began having thoughts or ideas that seemed to be cowboy related, so I asked about any stories she might remember with him about that. And then, I had an image of him, standing tall and handsome, smiling. At death, he was a paraplegic. I kept seeing him standing on rustic flooring with a long bar across the room. The rustic flooring and bar were symbolic to me of the West and of cowboy country. He let me know that his mom had to figure it out. And he was clearly having fun with this, with her, and with me. She did figure it out. The rustic flooring had replaced carpeting in his condo, and a long bar separated his kitchen from the den. His mother and two sisters would be spending the night there to celebrate him and the Fourth of July as he had celebrated with them six months prior. The sale of his condo was to close a few days later, but not before they knew that, in spirit, he would be joining them for another celebration.

There are times when after-death communication occurs in dreams or sleep-time awareness. A little more than two years after attending a former childhood friend's funeral and during the time I was writing this book, I was quite surprised to be visited during sleep by her. Though as adults we had been university colleagues, we had not seen or talked to each other in probably fifteen years. I was unable to discern any specific messages, but she continued to be fully present in my dream consciousness until I had clearly committed to myself, and I guess therefore to her, that I would find a way to contact her only child to tell her of the visit. I had no idea if her daughter would be receptive. It took a day and a half for me to find her and her telephone number in the neighboring state where she lived. I only knew that I would let her know that her mother had contacted me and stayed present until seemingly satisfied that I would call. My sense of that insistence was also to give loving assurance to her daughter, a woman in her forties with two children of college age. While gathering the contact information, I learned why my friend wanted so strongly for her daughter to receive her message of love: her father had died some years before; her mom, my friend, died in 2013 from cancer; several months later her maternal grandmother who lived nearby died; and just a few months before her mother's insistent appearance in my dream state, her husband had lost his life to a lengthy battle with cancer. In less than three years, she was orphaned and widowed. I had not known. How loving—how amazing—that a message of love survives to the end … and on.

Can I say with certainty that the message was fully received or fully believed? No. What I choose to say is that, at the very least, my reaching out and caring was a kind of surrogate love that the daughter, whom I had known as a young girl, did acknowledge. At the very least, my dream with her mother generated loving words and actions. Explain it any way you'd like; I'm comfortable with love beyond death.

The dying often have encounters with loved ones as they are leaving their bodies. Deathbed vision stories simultaneously are often after-death communication experiences, so much so that they are the subject of a chapter of their own. And they are awe-inspiring.

5

Visions

The young, inexperienced nurse simply did not know how to respond to her dying patient. The person he wanted to introduce—the one to whom he was talking and at whom he was smiling and nodding—was simply invisible to her. Hospice nurses Maggie Callanan and Patricia Kelley in their pioneering book, *Final Gifts,* tell us that the theme most prevalent in nearing-death awareness seems to be the presence of someone not alive. The timing may vary, sometimes happening hours, days, or even weeks before actual death. [21]

Near-death visions, nearing-death awareness, death-related sensory experiences, deathbed phenomena, deathbed apparitions, deathbed visions, and shared death experiences are all terms to describe what seems to be quite common. The place they occur and the time prior to death vary.

In the article "Deathbed Phenomena and Their Effect on a Palliative Care Team: A Pilot Study," Sue Brayne, Chris Farnham, MD, and Peter Fenwick, MD, reported that patients regularly share such phenomena as important in their dying process. Deathbed phenomena (DBP) were reported as comprising a far broader scope than only images of apparitions at the end of the bed. So important, so numerous were the patient reports of deathbed phenomena that the authors raised concerns about the need for training and education to help palliative care teams with the wider implications of their research results.[22] Their study also suggested many DBP may go unreported, are not drug-induced, and that patients may prefer talking to nurses rather than doctors about their experiences.

Various media sources, following the death of Steve Jobs in 2011, reported that his last words were: "Oh wow. Oh wow. Oh wow." Perhaps with a similar meaning, in 1931, Thomas Edison is said to have emerged from a coma hours before his death, opened his eyes, looked upward, and said, "It is very beautiful over there." And legend also has it that Ludwig van Beethoven, unable to hear in the last ten years of his life, said, when dying in 1827, "I shall hear in heaven!"

As you read this chapter, you can help yourself, family members, friends, or patients by becoming more familiar with what the dying may want to share with you. At first, you may simply need to accept that you may hear amazing things. For some, what you do with that acceptance could take more time, more reading, more experience, more evaluation … and more suspension of disbelief.

Dr. Karen Wyatt, a hospice medical director caring for patients in their homes, has written about a beautiful, soft light surrounding dying patients in their beds. She describes looking around for a source for the light until she became satisfied with what she recognized the light to be and explains what that might be.[23]

In 2005 and 2006, Marilyn A. Mendoza, PhD, surveyed nurses in Louisiana and Maryland. The last item in the survey was a blank page where the respondents were encouraged to write stories about their more memorable experiences with deathbed patients. She uses their reports to help us understand patient experiences as being of great importance among all the things happening when death nears. As an example, seeing a deceased relative or a beloved pet commonly brings both peace and comfort. She tells encouraging, loving, heartwarming deathbed stories in her book.[24]

Mistakes that nurses, doctors, and family members sometimes make include trying to talk dying persons out of what they say they have seen or heard, claiming the impossibility of such an occurrence, declaring that one or another type of medication is the cause, or simply ignoring the patient. A better path, which requires compassion, though no medical training, is listening and trying to understand both the meaning of the vision and its importance to the patient. It requires loving.

Just after seven in the morning, my phone rang, and from a city some 250 miles away. Through her tears, the caller said, "Lynn, this is Nancy. Mom's dying."

Her mom, Marie, was a friend with whom I had shared many unique experiences. Nancy reminded me that ten years before, her mom's physician had counseled her she might have only about five years to live; her lungs were that bad. We cried and talked together for a while. I sensed Nancy wanted reassurances about several things related to death and dying. So I mentioned some of the near-death visions that people have had of loved ones coming for them, and I mentioned some NDErs recounting reunions with loved ones who had predeceased them. Nancy wondered who might be there for her mom. "Her brother?" she asked.

I didn't sense him or Marie's mother. "I think her dad," I told her. "But they could all come."

In a text message the following morning, Nancy told me she and her mom had talked about some of the things we had discussed. "You were right," Nancy texted. "She told me that when she got out of the hospital last Christmas after being treated for pneumonia, the night she got home, she looked up on the closet door in her room and her dad was waving to her, sliding down a sliding board. She said she knew it wasn't time then, but it meant he would be back."

Anyone who hadn't known her dad, Lon, might think that a seriously ill Marie was hallucinating. But anyone who had known that big, gregarious, loving man who was adored by his daughter would laugh with them both at his playful message and appearance. In the hospital this time, Marie continued to hang on. Who could really know why? One could speculate, as I did, that her huge, loving heart wanted to continue to care for her husband of fifty-two years who had his own significant health issues.

Nancy later told me she saw her deceased uncle in the room and described "his smirk and loving eyes," and she sensed Pop, her grandfather. A cup of orange juice spilled unassisted from a wide-armed chair, and a small piece of hospital equipment fell from somewhere, hitting Nancy on the shoulder. Nancy was reassured, not spooked, that her uncle and grandfather were there, ready to assist her mom in transitioning. We are confident they did.

Psychiatrist Elisabeth Kübler-Ross, a pioneer in the examination and understanding of the death process, suggested that perhaps the best way to study and verify the dying person's awareness of deceased family or friends is to sit with dying children after family accidents. She would sit with them, watching silently, often holding their hands, and listen. They would sometimes name those preceding them in death. Dr. Kübler-Ross did not claim to know how to explain this.[25]

Dr. Allan J. Hamilton has written about multiple quasi-successful skin transplant surgeries on a burned young boy who remained in a coma, approaching death. The story includes the boy's surprising postsurgery description of a deceased relative he insisted was standing nearby.[26]

Frequently, death as a journey is a theme among the dying, and that theme is often presented in conjunction with a vision. The dying will ask if you have bought the bus, train, or plane tickets. They may ask if you have picked up a suit or dress from the cleaners, because they must get dressed to go. In one reported instance, a man said he must dress quickly because his driver had come to his room and let him know that his limousine was waiting.

A very elderly loved one nearing her end of life continuously cautioned her goddaughter, my friend Anna, that they really needed to hurry. Even though the destination was never specific, she was insistent they were going to be late.

Famous ballerina Anna Pavlova was especially remembered for her portrayal of a swan in *The Dying Swan* and in *Swan Lake*. With her last words, she is said to have asked to have her swan costume ready and to play the last measure softly.[27]

Marilyn Mendoza, PhD, describes a patient sitting up in bed, looking up at the ceiling in the corner of the room and talking to her sister as if she were in the room, though the sister had died ten years previously. Two days later, that patient died.[28]

Hospice nurse Janet Wehr tells the story of Lisa, who was completing the paperwork to admit Walt as a hospice patient when he apologetically asked her to leave. When she soothingly asked him if there was a reason, he explained that they had come for him.

Lisa leaned toward Walt and quietly asked him who had come. He extended his arm in the visually empty space to his left and lovingly identified his wife. And next, he extended his arm a bit more and reverently introduced "Our Lord."[29] Lisa left his room to file the paperwork, and when she returned, less than fifteen minutes later, Walt had died. Wehr also recounts many other stories of love.

Hospice physician Pamela Kircher recalls numerous incidents of predeath visions. In *Love Is the Link,* she explains that her hospice experience has taught her that visitations from dead relatives can be one of the ways of knowing that a person is entering into the final days of life.[30] She explains further that these visits bring great comfort.

Hospice nurses Callanan and Kelley suggest your best response is acceptance, rather than searching for other explanations for deathbed stories. They say you should also tell the truth. If you are told that a deceased loved one has been to visit and are then asked if you know where that person is, of course you can provide information about the person's death years ago, saying what you recall. It's best not to contradict; the dying knows what he has seen and his personal reality. You can ask to hear more about the visit and perhaps learn more.[31] The most important thing, and perhaps the most exciting, is to realize that when a dying person sees someone invisible to you, then death is not lonely. The stories the dying tell us are that they haven't died alone. If you can accept that, then you can take comfort in expecting that neither will you.[32]

Some of the visions also include out-of-body experiences, even travel; some were described as part of a near-death experience. Occasionally, a caregiver or family member may also participate in the OBE. My friend Bev, as noted in an earlier chapter, had that experience briefly with Reggie as he died.

6

Participation in Visions

Having personally had two near-death experiences, William Peters, MEd, MFT, founder of Shared Death Crossing Project, was witness in 1998 to his paternal grandmother's near-death visions and possible conversations with deceased relatives and friends. Later, in his hospice work, he learned that his grandmother's experiences are commonly referred to as predeath visions. He also found that they are routinely devalued in Western medical institutions as hallucinations.[33] For those experiencing or witnessing visions, they can be discouraged by having what is real to them discounted as a hallucination, and to do so is not to love, but to deny exquisite possibility. Fortunately, acceptance of such visions is increasing.

When family, nurses, and others experience or participate in a person's departure, it is a profound experience and, sometimes, an enormous opening to what truly may be possible. As a young nurse, Lea worked in a nursing home. When she arrived late one evening for the night shift, she noticed one of the patients seated in a dining area. Zelda was a lovely lady; her deceased husband had been a young bodyguard to the king of Norway during World War II. Concerned for Zelda, Lea approached her and offered to help her return to her room, explaining that it was too late for supper and too early for breakfast.

But Zelda told her she was fine and added, "Lisa said it is okay."

So Lea proceeded to the administrative area to check in, where she saw former army nurse Lisa, who was charge nurse for the night. Still concerned for Zelda, Lea told Lisa of their conversation in the dining area. But Lisa had surprising information. "Lea, Zelda died this morning, and her body has already gone to the funeral home."

Lea told me that to this day she wonders if she would have been able to physically feel Zelda if she'd reached out to touch her. She could see and hear her. Could she have felt her too?

Only a couple of years after her experience with Zelda, Lea's twenty-three-year-old sister was diagnosed with an autoimmune disease on a Thursday. Very quickly, her sister began bleeding out and was intubated. Communication was not possible. The following Tuesday, her sister died. Lea suffered deeply, crying almost incessantly and suffering intense headaches. She was mourning deeply. After two weeks had passed, Lea saw and felt her deceased sister sitting on the side of her bed. She remembers asking her sister what heaven is like. "Disneyland, only better," her sister said. After the visit, Lea continued to cry a lot, but her headaches were gone.

Though they may cling to the word *hallucinations*[34] rather than consider more radical possibilities, many studies have reinforced active communication between living spouses following the death of their mates. The research reports visual, audial, and tactile encounters. In studies of Welsh living spouses, about half of the widows and widowers tell of sensing the presence of their dead spouse. Sadly, up to 75 percent report never mentioning their experience to anyone else, even though the encounters were experienced as comforting. Though for most the experience occurs soon after the death of the spouse, there are many later appearances that have been described as a comfort, even though they occur years beyond the usual period of adjustment.[35]

For the six years since her death at age seventy-nine, in various ways, Nana has made herself known to her grandson Fred. She seems to enjoy being in her river home and finding ways to let others know she's there. Nana's heavy smoking had left that awful odor in her home, but it considerably lessened over time.

Two years after her death, Fred recalls going upstairs to the "rose room to fetch/look for something. As I opened the closed door, a heavy exhale of smoke was blown onto my face. The smell was easily recognizable as my grandmother's favorite cigarette, Pall

Mall. It never happened again. I'm thoroughly convinced this was my grandmother. I've convinced others too."

Fred also explains that his friends have experienced Nana, saying, "I've had close friends spend the night with me at the river [house] who've complained of being awakened at night to the playing of the upstairs piano. When showed the grandfather clock downstairs and asked if they could have gotten the two sounds mixed up, my friends quickly shake their heads and say, 'No.' Nana always loved playing 'Heart and Soul' on that piano."

Fred's sister Eve adds, "One of my friends and one of Fred's friends woke up at around what I would guess was 3 or 4 a.m. to the sound of 'Heart and Soul' being played on the piano. This happened on two different nights. I think it would be Nana playing the piano, because she always played 'Heart and Soul.' As far as I remember, it's the only song she played."

Some years later, Nana's physician husband was in an extended sleep, his body slowly shutting down. Two days before his death, he awakened for several hours and could be heard happily talking to his wife. Had she come to accompany him to a more ethereal home? His daughter, the mother of Fred and Eve, enthusiastically and appreciatively believes the answer is yes.

Betty and Jason adopted two male kittens, litter mates, naming them Max and Sam. They treated both kittens like children, though Max was especially affectionate with Betty. After Jason's death, Max became extremely attentive to Betty and began sleeping on her back with his head on her shoulder. Betty awakened one morning with Max lying on her back and stroking her hair with his front paw exactly the same way that Jason had done. Betty realized it was a totally unnatural motion for a cat to make with his leg and paw. It was also around this time that Betty had dreamed Jason told her, "Max is watching after you."

As their cat children exhibited other new behaviors, Betty decided to contact a reputed professional animal communicator, Miranda Alcott, to find out what Max's behavior was about. Without knowing any of the backstory, Betty recalls Miranda telling her, "Max says that Jason asked him to take care of you."

For some, beloved pets appear during waking hours. Having met a delightful young woman at a conference in Atlanta, Georgia,

I enjoyed conversing with her and hearing about her childhood in Ukraine before she emigrated to the United States more than twenty years previously. As I was listening to her talk about her relatives left behind and some sadness she still experienced when thinking about them, a dog came into my consciousness. The love of that dog for the young woman was so palpable that I became quite teary. As I described the dog and his love for her, she confirmed his being in her childhood and their mutual love and described the ways they had played together. In the act of describing, she brought those feelings of love back. Her physical countenance changed so markedly that some other attendees we knew nearby, without having been a part of our conversation, commented on how radiant she had become. Clearly, she and her long-deceased dog loved to the end … and on.

Over the years, I have had several conversations with my architect cousin Alice about the possibility of survival beyond the death of one's physical body. She had a very warm dimpled smile, twinkling eyes, and an adventuresome spirit. After she had been diagnosed with brain cancer, we speculated about how she might be able to let me know she was still around after her death. I explained that the butterfly is a frequently mentioned ADC sign, a spiritual symbol for life after death because of its metamorphosis from a ground-crawling caterpillar to something beautiful that flies free. After her death, when the family went to its remote private burial grounds, as prayers of thanksgiving for Alice began, a swarm of small yellow butterflies appeared. Not one, not two, but more yellow butterflies than we could count greeted us. Perhaps it was Alice telling us, "Hello, I'm here."

When my childhood friend Carrie was dying, drifting but still able to speak, she told her daughters that the bluebirds had come to get her and that she also saw Cotton (her recently deceased Bichon), and then she saw all of her earlier dogs and was so happy because the dogs were there. On the morning of her death, her younger daughter, Cindy, heard birds singing as she drove back to the house from the hospital; her granddaughter Ann felt and saw Carrie's presence on the end of her bed, and her daughter Ainsley's friend Lolly heard Carrie's laughter.

Queen of country singing Loretta Lynn has been remarkably open about her ability to both see and speak with friends and family who have passed on. She has described seeing her deceased friend Johnny Cash while she was recording in his old place, now the Cash Cabin Studio. Because they were such good friends, she has said she thought nothing of it until it suddenly hit her that she was seeing Johnny Cash in the studio; she quit singing.[36] The Cash vision was far from her first. She has discussed many other experiences in a lengthy YouTube interview with Glenn Eric: *Loretta Lynn's Haunted Plantation.*[37]

Midday on Friday, March 11, 2016, while speaking in California at the Reagan Library funeral of her mother, First Lady Nancy Reagan, Patti Davis remembered her mother's deep sense of loss when her father died. As I watched on television, Ms. Davis also recalled and shared her father's after-death visits, described by her mother as hearing the footsteps of her Ronnie coming down the hall and then having him sit beside her on the bed. Those visits of president Ronald Reagan to his beloved wife, she said, lasted for some time before they ceased. The following day in her weekly *Wall Street Journal* opinion piece, Ronald Reagan speechwriter Peggy Noonan wrote lovingly of President and Mrs. Reagan. And she echoed recollections of afterlife visions. Ms. Noonan recalled the first lady saying that she hadn't believed in the afterlife until things that happened after Ronnie died. He visited her. Mrs. Reagan said she could not explain it, but said that she had come to believe in the afterlife.[38]

Celeste struggled to move beyond her intense grief following the passing of her husband of fifty-eight years. Six months later, in an email to me and a group of others, she wrote of her continuing physical anguish. Even with admitted appreciation of her husband's death as a release from his intense pain, she remained agitated about conflicts concerning medical treatment, leaving the hospital so that he could die peacefully in their home, releasing his body for cremation, and her inability to obtain a properly signed death certificate, the latter resulting in her arrest. She recalled to us what saved her that first night was hearing her deceased husband speak to her as she was being arrested and his body removed: "Don't worry. I'm not there anymore. It's all right!" Her departing husband calmed her when she was confused and agitated by the professionals surrounding her. That memory sustains her as she recovers from feeling treated as an outlaw rather than as a loving spouse.

Sharing another unique family experience, the children, grandchildren, and even great-grandchildren of Norman, the eldest practicing attorney in Mobile, Alabama, at age ninety-seven, were gathered in both sadness and celebration after his death. One of his children, Sharon, had been among my closest friends and remained so. When I heard that her dad had died, I immediately baked some goodies to take by their childhood home where they were all gathered from various US cities. And knowing that they are very close-knit and probably wanting privacy to do what needed doing, I did not expect to stay but to briefly hug and postpone visiting until a later time. How shocked I was when whoever opened the door said, "Oh, Lynn, we're so glad you're here. Come in. We have some questions we just have to ask you. Someone, quick, go wake up Pete."

Pete, a grandson of Norman, is the son of Sharon's sister Olivia, who was still en route back to the United States from Russia and, sadly for all, was the only sibling not present. The other two, Martha and Edmund, were. Pete stumbled in sleepily from his interrupted nap and sat down among the gathered family. As so often over the years, I felt included as part of the family.

There was an intensity of feeling among everyone there. Once seated, Pete and Martha began asking questions and telling me things in a barrage of words. At the time of Norm's death, both of them had witnessed something neither thought was possible, and both had essentially the same experience, which is detailed in the following paragraph. To confound that surprise, the experience was in opposition to all they had been taught. Growing up in the traditions of Reform Judaism, often each had repeated the words, "The departed whom we now remember have entered into the peace of life eternal. They still live on earth in the acts of goodness they performed and in the hearts of those who cherish their memory. May the beauty of their life abide among us as a loving benediction. May the Father of peace send peace to all who mourn, and comfort all the bereaved among us."[39] What they had seen could not have been, but it was seen, at least to both of them. As Norm departed, so did their worldview as they had known it. I could not answer all their questions; they could not fully process even the questions they formed.

While writing this, I contacted the family for details and for purposes of accuracy. Pete has written to me with passion and specificity:

> It's wonderful that you are still helping people understand the mysteries that can occur at the end of one's life. It's been almost ten years since the passing of my grandfather, and the memories are still very clear. I'll recount those memories so they are communicated as factually as possible. In the last conversation I had with Grandad, he expressed his relief that my mom was out of the country. He stated that he felt experiencing his life ending would be too hard for her. Grandad's dying took several days. Throughout this time, my mom was doing everything in her power to get from Russia back to Mobile, Alabama. What she didn't realize was there were larger forces working against her. She experienced obscure visa issues, flights delayed for no reason, and finally, absolutely every flight into Mobile, Pensacola, or any other nearby town simply were canceled for no reason. In frustration, back in the United States, she called the family home in Mobile from the Atlanta airport and begged Grandad to hold on. Then she said, with all able to hear, "But if you can't hold on, it's okay for you to go." At that moment, my grandfather, who was down to one breath every ten seconds, opened his eyes. His body lurched upward as if he were reaching for something and simply popped out of his flesh. There was no smoke or spirit image of him, but the second before and the second after were like night and day. At this point, time changed. Seconds felt like hours. I looked over at my cousin, Ben, and saw an aura of energy surrounding him and had an immediate knowledge that he and all of us were going to be okay. At this moment, I also felt a sense of euphoria that is hard to

> describe. It was as if I stuck my pinky in eternity, and the sense of love and peace was beyond belief. My grandfather died at ten minutes before ten. I know this because all the clocks in the house stopped the exact moment of his passing. Further, when my sister, Eva, got back to her apartment in NYC, she called to tell me her clock had also stopped at this time.
>
> The events surrounding Grandad's passing were a gift. They revealed to me that there is something much bigger out there that we will all get to experience. It showed me that there is a force of energy that is so full of love and that we are all part of this and connected to it.
>
> For some in our family, the events of my grandfather's passing are viewed as personal and sacred. Because of this, when sharing the experience, we ask that you simply substitute names to honor the privacy of our family.

As a culture, we have inadequately prepared ourselves for the possibility of deathbed visions or shared death experiences. In *Glimpses of Eternity*, Raymond Moody, MD, writes that he didn't hear about the phrase *shared death experience* until the mid-1980s as doctors and nurses began telling each other deathbed stories. He realized, he says, that shared death experiences have always been with us, but doctors and nurses seemed to be discouraged from speaking about things considered spiritual and not scientific.[40]

Preliminary research from Shared Crossing Research Initiative and Dr. Moody's research indicate there may be many benefits from shared death experiences. These include, but are not limited to, grief reduction, increasing awareness and belief in a possible afterlife, less fear of death, and a refocusing on and deepening understanding of purpose in one's life.[41]

Another kind of vision also occurs for both the dying and their loved ones. They encounter what they believe to be, for lack of another culturally shared word, angels.

In reading *The Rotarian*, December 2015, I was thrilled to learn about a billionaire philanthropist born in a poor, black neighborhood in Tuscaloosa, Alabama. His remarkable life story includes the time when he was seriously ill as a toddler, and two angels mysteriously appeared in the form of white women in long dresses who hurriedly directed his father to a doctor across town who could and did treat him. The women quickly left and were never seen again. His family believes God sent them to spare his life and to show that God had a purpose for him. He maintains that his faith has been the foundation for his success and philanthropy and that he can still sense the presence of his ladies, his life-saving angels.[42]

Reading about the philanthropist, I remembered the story a friend told me many years ago—years and years before cell phones existed. It wasn't a deathbed story. It could have been. Fred was a big guy with multiple talents. He was funny and kind, and without pretension. He was bilingual. Among other professions, Fred had experience as a faith leader and as a cartoonist. At one time, Fred decided to paint the interiors of new houses. On one job, he was the lone painter inside the home with doors and windows closed. Whatever paint he had been asked to use created fumes noxious enough that Fred realized he was in trouble. He remembered falling, unable to reach an exit door. His next memory was lying on the ground in the fresh air outside that house, opening his eyes, and seeing two people disappear. No one else was around, no one knew Fred had been alone in that house, no one knew he had passed out in a closed house, and yet, someone rescued him from that ill-fated environment, dragging him to safety. At first, when he opened his eyes and saw two people leaving, a man and a woman, he thought possibly they might be the owners of the house he had been painting. After the event, Fred believed and maintained that they were angels. There really was no logical explanation for their presence or his rescue.

Many people who have found themselves to be in a perilous situation return to tell stories of someone being with them and sustaining them. There are instances where trapped miners have barely survived and have given credit to a being who appeared in the mine with them to give courage and comfort. Hunters have told stories of getting lost in the woods and then becoming aware of another hunter ahead of them who remained always just ahead until they regained safety, only to have the elusive hunter-guide disappear completely. There are stories of mountain climbers who have fallen or who began suffering from hyperthermia, who, for varying reasons, credit their survival to the presence of another being. Pilots flying solo often speak of sensing a copilot in the plane, one who is sometimes credited with a miraculous course correction or safe landing. Are they delusional? Given that, in group situations, more than one person gives the same descriptions, it is difficult to say that each is experiencing the same delusion. In traditional religious literature, the presence of such beings may be credited to a guardian angel. In more secular literature, such a presence may be attributed to what some call the third man.

These stories are enough reason to strengthen our conversations. Embrace possibilities. Share our experiences. Suspend our disbeliefs. It is time we love enough to honor the impossible when we feel its embrace.

Sometimes, the incredibly, impossibly possible comes both before and after death. Sometimes, we answer the call to love while dying and delight in sharing that love again, even years after death has occurred.

7

Allowing Life, Death, and Love to Lead

On that January Thursday in 2003, the phone rang only once.

"Good morning."

"Hello, Lynn? This is Tom."

"Hi, Tom!" I said with a hint of surprise and a great deal of pleasure in my voice.

"Lynn, I'm here in the hospital room with Hugh [Tom's brother], and he wants to talk to you. Okay?"

I answered enthusiastically. "Yes, of course."

Some noises and a female voice, a nurse or technician if judged by sound, were audible in the background. A pause followed. So I asked, "Tom, is this something to do with remission?" I was thinking the word *reoccurrence* in reference to leukemia, but instead, I used the word *remission*.

"No," Tom said. "He'd like to see you. Let me give you this phone number. Do you know how to get here?"

"No."

Tom gave me the hospital name and phone number, Hugh's room number, and directions to the hospital in a city about sixty miles away in a neighboring state.

"Are you sure Hugh wants me there, Tom? You know how he is."

"Things are different now. Here's Hugh."

"Hello."

"Hello?" Hugh responded.

"Hello," I repeated.

"Hello? I can't hear her."

"Put that up to your ear, Hugh. No, Hugh, up to your ear." It was Tom's voice.

Unease and sadness began their journey into my being. Again, I heard Hugh's voice, a little raspy and low, "Hello?"

"Hi, Hugh."

"Lynn, I want to apologize to you for not being better about staying in touch. I'm sorry I haven't been a better friend."

"Hugh, you've no need to apologize."

"You're a wonderful person." It was his voice and not his voice.

Smiling ever so slightly and using a tone of teasing humor, I said, "And you too, Hugh. Would you like me to come over there?"

"Yes."

"Good. I'll try to get over there soon." I sensed Hugh's effort at conversing. "Could I speak to Tom again?"

"Yes. Lynn?"

"Tommy, I'll be there, but I don't think I can make it before the weekend. Will that be okay?"

"That'll be fine."

"Okay, I'll see you then."

The phone rested in its cradle only a few minutes, just long enough to ruminate briefly. I had not known that Hugh was in the hospital. I reflected on the tone and content of the unexpected conversation.

My fingers quickly tapped out the phone number of a good friend who knew Hugh and his family well. After just a couple of rings, she answered. "Hello?"

"Anna, Tom just called me from Hugh's hospital room. Hugh wants me to come over. He sounds really sick this time. I don't—"

Cutting in, she said, "I know; they thought a few days ago he wasn't going to make it."

"I didn't know he was seriously sick again."

"Oh yes, I think he went to the hospital last Friday or Saturday," Anna explained.

Anxiety began to set in, a hint of pain affecting my speech. "I told Tommy I didn't think I could get there before the weekend."

"Do you think you really want to wait?"

"I don't know how I can get there. I have more people I'm interviewing to take care of Dad and appointments and—"

"You've had so much going on with your Dad and now this. It's a lot. You don't need this now."

Having looked at my watch as she was speaking, I interrupted. "You know what, Anna … If I go right now, I just may be able to get there. Bye."

I dialed the hospital phone number, requested to be connected with Hugh's room number, and Tom's voice answered. "Hello?"

"Tom, hi, this is Lynn. Tom, I have this window of opportunity, and I'll be there in the early afternoon, even if it's only for about ten minutes."

"Okay, we'll see you then."

"Tom, is there anything he needs or anything you'd suggest that he might enjoy?" I asked.

"No, just come on over."

Fast-forward through several things that had to be done. Behind the wheel of my Olympic-blue Audi Allroad, I realized that travel was easy and traffic lighter than expected. The sky was clear, and the sun was shining brightly—a beautiful, crisp day. My mind wandered back to Hugh's first words on the phone: "I want to apologize." And my response that he didn't need to do that. I felt awful. I had refused what he felt a need to give. What a put-down. I was disappointed in myself for the inability to have said a simple, more loving, "Thank you."

About two-thirds of the way there, in the atmosphere of the car, I experienced a change of energy, a sense of someone from long ago—Hugh's mom. She had died when we were in high school.

"Let Hugh know I love him. Let him know I'm near." I more sensed than heard this.

Refocusing on the road, the trip went easily, as the directions I had were excellent. I stopped to buy flowers and a card, carefully choosing each.

The parking at the hospital appeared problematic. "Okay, God, guardian angels, someone show me where to drive to park." I made a turn and then another when I spotted a car backing out, vacating a legitimate space.

I walked through the entry lobby, down a hall, and along another long hall where I waited at an elevator to go up a floor. After walking down one more hall, I saw his room number and then a sign on the door that read: "Knock before entering."

My knuckles tapped on the door. "It's Lynn."

"Come in."

"Hi," I said, handing Tom the lavender-purple potted flowers. "There's a card you can read to Hugh later." I scanned the signs of concern visible in the room—the balloons, the flowers, and the small teddy bear attached to the side of the hospital bed.

Walking around the bed, I leaned over and kissed Hugh on his cool, clammy forehead, being careful not to touch the oxygen mask covering his nose or jiggle the stand that held bags dripping liquids into his IV. "Hi, Hugh."

Opening his eyes, Hugh said with somewhat strained, muted voice, "I want to apologize, Lynn, for not being more in touch."

"I appreciate that, Hugh. Friends like us stay friends, and it's okay."

A barely visible nod of agreement was accompanied by a sound.

"Lynn, would you like to sit over here?" Tom asked.

"I'd like to be close enough to hold Hugh's hand. I'd rather sit over there."

Back around to the other side of the bed, sitting in the chair pulled close to the side of the bed, I reached over to take Hugh's hand. Hugh's head rested on two pillows. His eyes were closed, and his skin looked pale. His eyes fluttered with brief focus in my direction.

Sitting by my recumbent friend, holding hands, summoning courage, I said, "Hugh, you know how sometimes I hear and know things in ways some people don't? Well, on the way over here, I felt your mom in my car, and she wanted me to tell you how much she loves you."

Without opening his eyes, he said, "That's a nice thing to say." His succinct response was reflective of his tolerance of me, but also his guarded acceptance of my experience.

"Well, I sure didn't expect that, but you know that happens to me sometimes—like we talked about after you read my book about intuition and psychic stuff. Would you like to talk about any of those kinds of things?"

Not surprisingly, the answer was no. I knew this because he opened an eye and inquired about my family, one by one—every member of my family. He even asked about my father-in-law, who he had never met but with whom he shared the experience of leukemia.

A few moments of quiet passed. Hugh took his hand from mine to scratch his other hand and then reached out and took my hand again. His brows would knit; breathing would be all that he did for a bit.

"Hugh, the leukemia's really done a number on you this time, huh?"

"It really has," he responded in a barely audible, strained voice.

Quiet resumed. We continued to be there together, holding hands, content in the silence. Hugh appeared to have dozed off.

I asked Tom if Hugh knew about Dunc, a childhood friend of ours who had died a few weeks earlier. Again, Hugh opened his eyes slightly and asked about her, wanting to know and to comment. Tom asked about her older brother, his friend.

Tom and I talked about friendship briefly. We also found reasons for a little laughter and for appreciation of the joys of brotherhood. Hugh listened without comment.

A cleaning person came in to mop the floor. I lifted my feet and then stood. Again, I leaned over to kiss Hugh's forehead, which was still a bit cool and damp. I sat down again, and we held hands again. Tom talked about how Hugh had gone for a ride in a wheelchair that morning and commented on how proud he was of Hugh. The cleaning lady commented that Hugh was resting peacefully.

A glance at my watch showed that ten minutes had stretched to almost thirty, maybe more. I wasn't sure exactly. "I'm going to have to go now." I stood. "Hugh, I'm going to try to get back this weekend."

"I'm looking forward to it." He spoke quietly with eyes closed.

"Hugh, is there *anything* I can do for you?"

Eyes opening slightly, he looked at me. "You can be my friend."

"Hugh, I am your friend. I always have been, and I always will be." For the last time, I leaned over and kissed Hugh's forehead. "I love you."

Quietly, with his eyes closed, he spoke from beneath his oxygen mask. "I love you too."

They were words we'd never shared before—words to cherish always.

Tom stood and accompanied me from the room.

The drive home was easy. The emotions were not. I thought about taking a couple of books with me when I went back on the weekend—books Hugh had mailed to me from Princeton when we were in college and I had kept. I thought maybe I could just sit and read to him from works he had particularly liked. I wondered if I would have the chance. My stomach felt tight. My heart felt heavy.

Approaching the city limits, I called Anna on my cell phone. When prompted to leave a message, I rambled on. "He's really sick," I finally said and hung up.

There were a couple of things I needed to do for my dad, and then I had to be at his house to interview a potential home-health-care provider. Arriving at his house, I learned that the interviewee had called to say she would be late. Bummer. I wanted to get through the interview, go home, and sort through what I was thinking and feeling. And I wanted to get supper started for my husband and me.

I left for home to do some of that and to return to Dad's later. Unlike my usual procrastination, I checked for landline phone messages immediately—as soon as I was in the house. There were five messages. The first four were short.

The fifth had been recorded at about four thirty that afternoon. "Lynn, this is Tom. Hugh [not clear] at about three [not clear]. I'll let you know about what comes next. Thank you so much for coming over."

The bottom of my stomach disappeared. My whole body felt strange. What had I heard Tom say? Had he said Hugh died at 3:55? No, that couldn't be.

With trembling fingers, I searched for the paper on which I had written the hospital phone number. I called and asked for Hugh's room. No one answered. I hung up and called the hospital again. I explained that I'd had a phone call from the brother of a friend who was a patient there and asked to speak to the nurses' station closest to the room. Someone answered and listened to my request to speak to Tom and who he was.

"Just a moment," came the response. The music playing as I was on hold was of no comfort.

Another person came on the line. I gave the same explanation again. Time seemed to drag interminably. Eventually, another voice told me I would be connected.

"To the room?" I asked.

"No, to the location where the family is."

I had heard it. I had not wanted to hear what I heard.

"Hello?"

"Tom, this is Lynn. I couldn't clearly understand the message you left. Did you say that Hugh died at 3:55?"

"No, he died at 3:15. It was fifteen or twenty minutes after you left. He told me he'd like me to help him walk a little. He'd taken a few steps. He started having a hard time with his legs. I said, 'I better help you sit on the chair in the bathroom (the closest chair).' But I couldn't support him, and he just slid to the floor. He died very peacefully."

Numbness overcame me, as well as a very full feeling in my throat. The reason I felt numb could be attributed to many things. I had loved my friend—more about that later. I respected my friend. I would miss my friend and be eternally grateful for his final act of friendship. He was a special person to me, and he's worth your knowing more.

Hugh was a bit shy and average to above average in everything except golf and brains. In those, he was clearly ahead of the pack. By the time he was a teenager, Hugh was about five feet, ten inches tall; medium build; very regular features with short, sandy-colored hair; smooth, clear skin; and piercing blue eyes. It was easy to underestimate him.

Hugh knew this about himself, accepted it, and kept on quietly but confidently, excelling in his high school classes and on the golf course. His Latin teacher had asked him, "Hugh, have you mailed applications to college?"

"Yes, ma'am," he replied.

"And where have you applied?"

Without bravado, using an emotionless tone of voice reserved for statements of fact, he replied, "Harvard, Princeton, and Yale."

Hugh liked to think that life could continue to be fun. He was seventeen and the stalwart of his high school golf team. He also gave the adults in the championship league at The Country Club of Mobile a slim chance to win when he was on the links. Hugh's demeanor, modest size, and youthful, peach-skinned face often seduced the older golfers into delusional cockiness. At the age of ten, Hugh had won his flight in the Alabama State Junior Golf Tournament and, ceaselessly, had kept on getting better.

The Labor Day Invitational at the club was the competitive event of the year. Golfers came from around the country. A reputedly excellent adult golfer from Birmingham, Alabama, drew an early tee time and Hugh as his first-round opponent. The night before the tournament began Mr. Excellence was observed drinking at the bar. A friend commented that perhaps he should be getting a good night's sleep, to which he replied, laughingly, "No need to do that. My opponent's just a kid."

"Who's that?" the friend asked.

"Don't know him. Name's Hugh."

"Well then," his friend laughed, "you might as well start packing your suitcase to go home now."

As prophesied, Hugh, the kid, sent him home.

In classes, just as unobtrusively, Hugh brought in winning scores. He had been inducted into the National Honor Society in his junior year and given other honors too. He didn't do it the easy way, taking all the math, Latin, and science he could schedule.

Hugh didn't do parties and dating the easy way either. He was way too shy. He really didn't know how to make mindless conversation. He wasn't obsessed with Fats Domino, Shirley and Lee, or any of the emerging rock 'n' roll greats, but most of his classmates were. It wasn't that he didn't like popular music—he did. Hugh was just more comfortable in class and on the golf course than at a sock hop, dancing with the girls.

In his senior year, only a few months before his eighteenth birthday in January 1956, the strongest of Hugh's foundations was taken away. His mother died.

It was easy to tell that Hugh was deeply shaken. What was eating away at him inwardly began to show outwardly. The neat, soft-spoken, polite, friendly, young gentleman became increasingly quiet. His shirt was often untucked on one side, but in on the other.

His socks didn't match, sometimes not even his shoes. Hugh didn't notice, but his friends did.

Hugh was prepared for class, but there was a disorganization, even a randomness, to his work. His intense attentiveness in class often gave way to an uncharacteristic dreaminess—a glazed look at nowhere in particular. Even though his final grades would determine college acceptance, Hugh gave the appearance of having lost focus.

A clear speech pattern took on an occasional stutter. Hugh laughed less frequently. His habit of jauntily holding his chin up and a little to the side all but disappeared. But he never lost his kindness or his concern for others. Perhaps that was why he could still function at all.

With his father, older brother, and younger sister, Hugh continued to attend the Episcopal church regularly. He found solace in its rituals. He reinforced the memory of his mother's love with his favorite hymn, singing, "Jesus loves me, this I know, 'cause the Bible tells me so."

Gradually, Hugh began to get more of a grip on day-to-day living. He was learning to dig deeply within to a private reservoir of strength. Looking back, it was the beginning of his journey to a series of Walden Ponds where later he would choose to live in semisolitude.

His senior year in high school, however, was not a time he spent alone. Hugh was a member of a fraternity that did a few acts of charity and more of camaraderie. There were fraternity parties and dances, as well as school activities. He participated in most of them.

Hugh was genuinely well liked. He helped friends do classwork that baffled them but not him. He was sweet to everyone, but not the sissy, prissy kind of sweet. He simply didn't have a mean bone in his body. Sarcasm and gossip that were the mainstays of many teens were an anathema to Hugh. It was almost as though pettiness was beneath his personal radar. The loss of his mother accentuated his innate goodness. No one knew exactly why—then or ever.

When the class yearbook came out in the spring of 1956, no one, except perhaps Hugh himself, was surprised to see his picture featured as a senior notable. The description read: "Inspiration and genius, one and the same."

The question of college remained. Early admissions were not

an accepted practice in the fifties. Everyone waited. Hugh's friend Stanford was accepted to Harvard, his friend Barnes to Birmingham Southern, and his friend Bob to Georgia Tech.

And Hugh? Had the difficulties of his senior year affected his last semester grades required for final admission to the schools he'd chosen? Had he found the strength he needed to persevere? Somehow, the young boy becoming man had kept on doing what had to be done. He would not let his mother down; he would not let himself, his family, his friends, or his teachers down. He was accepted at Harvard, Princeton, and Yale. Hugh chose Princeton, where, four years later, in 1960, he completed a bachelor of science degree.

Hugh never married. He was devoted to his brother and sister and their children. He lived alone, sometimes hermit-like. He remained an avid reader. Some years he would send my husband and me flowers at Christmas and then be silent for a few years only to send flowers again. But he did not remain silent after he was no longer in his physical body—after he had died.

Nine years later, in 2012, I had a dream about Hugh. Not really about him, more with him. Though I have had lucid dreams where I can enter them, participate in them, and even change things around, this was different. The dream was more as though I was with him than I was dreaming about him. Usually, I can remember details of dreams about which I am aware. When I awakened, I could not remember specifics, but I had a sense that, together, we'd been to metaphysical night school, because other than intense love, all I could remember is something like: Anger can be sufficiently intense to burn itself up. Love is indestructible.

As I awakened more fully, the intense feelings about the nature of love, of love itself, stayed with me so strongly that I moved closer to my husband and stayed there, even skipping my early-morning trip to exercise. The sense of the dream as put into words is really inadequate. I wish I could help you to experience the feelings of that remarkable dreamtime visit. It has been an impetus to reach out to friends here and elsewhere with whom I have learned love through loving ... Now, that includes you.

Across our many years of friendship, I do not remember saying to Hugh, "I love you," or having him say those words to me. We did on the day he died.

In the words Hugh so often said in church, "Thanks be to God."

The day after Hugh's death, a very good friend and golf buddy of his called me, trying to make sense of it all, trying to soften his sadness. A former minister of a different faith, he had been asked to speak at Hugh's funeral and was struggling with that. I told him, and he repeated in the church, "Hugh was a teacher and taught us a life of introspection is not only lived in a monastery. He showed us self-respect and living from one's own directions can be compassionate and powerful. He allowed us to see one does not have to live up to societal norms and expectations but to live the love of creation."

Nine years after Hugh left his physical body, he continued his teaching in that most amazing dream visit, leaving a profound message for us now: *Anger can be sufficiently intense to burn itself up. Love is indestructible.*

And love occurs in many different ways, in the here and now … and on.

8

Bits of Laughter, Tears, and Love

In her last months, my ninety-two-year-old grandmother, Bobbie, wanted to eat only ripe bananas and chocolate candy. The competent staff in the care facility where she was being treated with great kindness complained to our family that they could not get her to eat sensibly. Though no one is ever sure about the timing of passage, of dying, we were fairly certain she had months left, if that. We laughed and said that bananas and chocolate candy made great sense to us, and from then on, that is what she ate—that is, when she even wanted to eat.

There was a Pillsbury refrigerated bakery goods advertisement many years ago that touted baked things from the oven being equated with lovin'. In my Bobbie's case, we loved her with bananas and chocolate. I still smile when I think of that.

About the time of my father's last hospitalization, either just before or after, we had encouraged his home caregivers to listen closely to his needs and be certain he was comfortable. Each day, he awakened fairly early, had breakfast, was up a short while before his morning nap, then had lunch, followed not long after by an afternoon nap, after which he would be up for a short while before his evening bourbon, then supper, and shortly after that to bed for the night.

One morning, when he first awakened, he said to his morning caregiver, "That was a really good nap. It must be time for my toddy.

Dad's late-afternoon routine included a bourbon and water that he sipped slowly before having his supper; he looked forward to it. The caregiver caught the phrase and realized Dad thought it was afternoon. Good for her. And without missing a beat, she asked, "Is that what you want?" After helping him to the bathroom, she brought him his drink, and then she fixed his supper—rather than his usual breakfast. He was happy and later went back to bed for a good night's sleep. When the replacement caregiver came, she was told the story. When Dad next awakened just before lunch, the exact same sequence occurred, as it did again at the normal supper time. We were delighted! He had eaten and slept well and was comfortable and happy—three bourbon and waters, three suppers. It's interesting to note that particular confusion was never repeated. But when it happened, he had been given loving care. Not arguments or corrections—just love.

The dying often breathe through their mouths. Hospice nurses usually explain to families how to use glycerin swab sticks for moistening the mouth, tongue, gums, or lips. Some are even lemon flavored. But some families have chosen instead to dip swab sticks into their loved one's favorite beverage. For my father, that would have been bourbon, if we had thought to do it.

"I don't want anyone to see me without my makeup," Carrie told her daughters from her hospital bed. Her hairbrush was gently used and makeup carefully applied by her daughters during the hours of her last days. Hearing being the last of the senses to go, surely she could share their happiness in the teasing they did of each other as they enjoyed for the last times doing girl things with their momma and loving her and each other in that special way.

In *Peaceful Passages*, Janet Wehr, RN, tells the story of a gentleman who required a urinary catheter greeting a new hospice nurse. She told him she would be changing the catheter. As soon as she pulled up his hospital gown, she heard him muttering about people calling men's genitalia privates. He declared his should be called his publics. They had a good laugh![43]

During her mother's final hours, my friend Venessa sat by her mother's bed and held her hand. When Venessa began singing one of her mother's favorites, she felt their love when her mom, no longer able to talk, squeezed her hand. She can still feel that last special physical sharing of love.

Maw-maw was approaching her one hundredth birthday. With a touch of the flu, her body weakened quickly. Within days, the family had gotten a hospital bed for her, and hospice help had been arranged. Her decline hastened. Family gathered around. One granddaughter told me they played Maw-maw's favorite gospel songs. As Elvis sang "How Great Thou Art," no longer able to speak and only a few hours from departing her body, Maw-maw lifted her hands and moved them in time to the music—"like she could see the rapture," laughed her lovingly amused granddaughter.

Declaring that our births and deaths are, perhaps, the two most important frames of life, a physician described in a *Wall Street Journal* article how his team assisted a family in honoring a loved one's deathbed request for submersion baptism. The team arranged for an inflatable pool to be filled in the ICU, first using a bucket brigade and then rigging a dialysis tube to circulate a stream of warm water. Then a patient-transfer lift lowered the patient, his ventilator temporarily unplugged, into the pool where his baptism occurred. The patient came out smiling. A palliative care social worker sang "Amazing Grace."[44]

An email let me know that a mutual friend was in intensive care in a local hospital. Sixty-five-year-old Ted had called out to his wife, "I can't breathe!" She called 911. He said later he felt as though he were suffocating. He remembered little after the paramedics arrived or through his ten days in cardiac intensive care at a nearby hospital where he was intubated, machines breathing for him. He was later told that his lungs, swollen with fluids, were strangling his heart. His heart stopped twice; he died twice. Both times he was resuscitated. He was moved to a private room and remained comatose and unresponsive, only exhibiting brief responsiveness a couple of times.

A physician suggested identifying some kind of stimulation to bring Ted fully back. His wife turned to Ted's lifelong friend Morris, who on some visits had left crying, fearing Ted was not going to recover. Morris had visited him often. A fellow amateur radio operator, Morris put a stimulation plan into action, returning to Ted's room with a handi-talkie (handheld radio). Morris began talking very loudly to him by his call letters. Then he put his fingers in Ted's hand, saying, "If you can hear me, squeeze my hand." Feeling his hand being squeezed, Morris began speaking even more loudly, proclaiming success.

He excitedly set up the radio and charging unit on a shelf and left to contact other amateur radio folks, telling them that Ted would be listening but be unable to speak. Using an emergency practice net fortunately scheduled for that night, person after person after person began loudly contacting Ted by his call letters and his name, wishing him well for a speedy recovery. He did regain consciousness. He could neither move nor speak, but he could produce tears and feel them streaming down both cheeks.

After hospitalization, he learned of the prayer groups and chains that had been formed on his behalf, composed of family members, friends, and the many ham operators worldwide who were praying for him. He learned of requests for prayer in church bulletins of several denominations. He professed his gratitude to them all. He has said to me, "I firmly believe that those prayers are the reason that I am here today. Prayers really work." As this was written months later, Ted had not fully recovered but was well on his way.

A highly intuitive person, former Silva Method instructor, and law-related professional, Ted had always been open to anomalous or mystical experiences. He acknowledged that, since dying twice, he feels, as I have when near him, that he has a crowd surrounding him at all times: a crowd of loved ones no longer in physical bodies or perhaps of angels assigned to assist him in his healing and the work here he has left to do. His return from death, he said, has made him even more spiritual, more convinced of the power of prayer, and more appreciative of fully living for what lies both ahead … and, eventually, on.

Molly recalled that her last cherished, memorable time with her mom, Emily, was actually the weekend before she passed. She had driven from Knoxville, Tennessee, to Louisville, Kentucky, on Friday night and planned to stay until Monday morning. Emily had some chores for her to do, running some errands and taking cookies to a neighbor. She recalls her mom always thinking about others before herself.

Molly had brought the next-door neighbor's kids a gingerbread house to build. Emily was thrilled; she wasn't able to get them a gift, but this was perfect in her eyes. Over the weekend, she wanted Molly to help her gather gifts for the family since Hanukkah was quickly approaching. Doing so filled the weekend with buying the gifts Emily wanted to share with their family. By Sunday, they had managed to get the job done together. Everyone had a gift. At her mom's request, Molly even wrapped the calendar Emily was giving her. Little did they know her mom would pass away three days later. Molly still has that calendar wrapped up and says, "I will keep it forever because it was a gift from Mom's heart to mine."

Webster was a big honeypot of a man with a great laugh and kind eyes. He was strong, adventuresome, and in his sixties. He had a history of heart problems and a probable limited life expectancy. When he had married Sandra, not the first marriage for either, he told her he hoped for ten years but realistically expected five. In February he had a stroke. Together, they looked forward to their usual summer boating activities. In May, he fell off a dock, breaking two ribs. Also in May, Sandra blew the boat's engine, and into repair it went. There was more than enough tension. Sandra commented to Webster that they were great at being lovers, not so good as patient and nurse. In early September, Webster brought home the repaired boat, tied it to the dock, and said to Sandra when she met him at their dock, "Come on, get in; we need to go make love."

Given his recent illnesses, she asked, "Are you kidding, or are you serious?"

With his assurances, she excitedly rushed back in the house to change into something sexy. Sandra assured me they thoroughly enjoyed each other, letting the boat all but drive itself. Several days later, they again enjoyed lovemaking. A few days later, Webster tucked Sandra in bed for the night, kissed her, and went to another room; somewhat of an insomniac, he often wandered around until late. Just after four in the morning, Sandra awakened to what sounded like snoring and then different than snoring. At four thirty, she heard the death rattle and ran to find him where he was lying in another bed, unresponsive and with his eyes half open. She called some nearby workers, who rushed over and did CPR until the ambulance came. Resuscitation was impossible. Just the day before, he had been splitting logs for Sandra for the outdoor fire pits she loved, another way he was loving her ... while he could.

Sandra is convinced Webster knew death was near. Indeed, it was the five years he had guesstimated. Webster's son told Sandra, "I always knew he was gonna be like an ole dog, just walk off in the woods and die."

She says, "The soul knows what the body doesn't."

Twice since Webster's physical death, a worker has seen him in the house. Sandra has sensed his presence and continues to feel his love.

In Ohio, Jim's anxious wife stood by his bed, a hospice nurse with her. Jim had been in serious decline, his body slowly shutting down. The nurse whispered encouragingly to his wife, helping her to speak to him, to say the words of release.

Anna tensed, saying softly through her tears, "It's okay, Jim. It's okay to go now."

Startled, Anna and the nurse heard, "Thank God!" as Jim sprayed urine all over them and the room. Shock and laughter ruled. And throughout the hospice itself, laughingly, word spread: "When the time comes, it's best to tell a man he can leave. Do not use the word *go*!"

Jim died not long after.

Raven, a woman not known for offhand or effusive statements of love to visitors, was being treated for end-stage cancer in her local hospital. Through blinding snow and over icy roads, friends and family visited. To their shock, surprise, and delight, Raven reached out to each of them and said, "I love you." Her breathing became labored, and her eyes were more closed than open. Raised in the Roman Catholic church, she had not been a church-going, practicing Catholic in many years, but she asked for a priest to come and administer last rites. Those who cared most encircled her bed, staying connected and hoping she could feel their love. In the early evening before her death the following midday, Raven rapidly raised her arms upward and loudly said, "Wahoo!" What a joyful parting gift.

Having joyful things to think about is helpful. We all know, though, that we have many times when tears are helpful too. Tears can release feelings, can be eye lubricants, and can sometimes remove stress or improve moods. They do not erase the reason we are sad, but they clear the path to remember our joy—our love.

Through the laughter and the tears, we cope. We do the best we can. There are ways we might do better and be more comfortable. If we have some tools and ideas for improving on guessing rather than simply reacting, we have a better chance to be proactive.

9

Managing to Make Better Decisions to the End … and On

Those last six months with my father were full of both wonders and atrocities. If I had only thought to use more of what I know, maybe everyone could have been more comfortable. The outcome might have been no different at all, but the process may have been decidedly less hurtful. We had lots of love, but sometimes there was not enough joy. I can only tell you the story of what happened and give suggestions about what might have made things better. I cannot change what we did, but in the telling, I hope you find ways to make wiser decisions and better choices and to have more moments of cheerful love.

My family ceded almost all our father's health management decisions to health-care professionals. We tacitly agreed that medical decisions overrode others. Maybe that was a mistake. There were more issues, peripheral ones, and many of those included additional caregivers and advisors. Maybe if we had thought in terms of better managing of people and processes, we might have had more joy to the end … and on.

Let me attempt to explain what I mean. Think about your favorite play or movie. You remember the plot, the action, and the dominant characters. But with your really favorite ones, you often remember most passionately the scenery, the ambiance, or a particular scene.

Something small or incidental touches you and gets into your innermost thoughts and feelings.

Similarly, that would be managing those things that are not part of a prescribed medical plan or treatment, but things that happen in support of the patient and the family and are crucial to the comfort and well-being of all. You may do the managing, or you may be part of a team assembled by someone who has taken on that role. That someone, acting as leader, can shift as needs and talents require.

I have previously written of one particularly satisfying occurrence. Very near his end of life, my dad had a day when he awakened in the morning after a brief morning nap, and after his usual afternoon nap, each time thinking that it was afternoon and time for his early evening toddy of bourbon and water, which he sipped before eating his supper. His caregivers recognized his confusion but did not increase it by trying to correct him. And that day he had three evening cocktails followed by three suppers—no breakfast or lunch foods. He was well-nourished and happy. That particular confusion was never repeated. All of us felt better because his peripheral, nonmedical needs had been heard and met in the moment. No one had contradicted him; no one had made him feel bad about his confusion. Individual situations were peripherally managed … one caregiver, one team management member as momentary leader at a time.

So, if you are involved in management, just what is it that managers do? In regard to whatever is being managed, you answer the questions: Who? What? When? Where? How/in what ways? And you answer them for any number of issues. By substituting "in what ways" for "how," you will increase your options.

Now-deceased famous author, management consultant, and Harvard professor Peter Drucker simplifies what is essential for management effectiveness: managing time, choosing what you can contribute, knowing where and in what ways to best mobilize strength, setting the right priorities, and weaving them all together with good decision-making. Dr. Drucker has suggested that management is also deeply involved in spiritual concerns—the nature of man, good and evil. It follows, then, that you'll need to focus on knowledge, on effectiveness, and on results, especially, but not limited to, a sick patient, and you'll need to expand your ideas of physical healing to a more encompassing one. Your decisions may be more about what works for the patient and the family's body-mind-spirit than about what treatment has the best odds for physical results. And, when end of life is apparent, using hospice services may sensitively assist with figuring out a managerial path and process—one that might feel to you as though it is just beyond rational thought, just beyond your grasp. And it will be a path that often expands to ideas beyond the purely physical ones.

Given that you will be making management decisions, even if only peripherally, a clearer, more specialized understanding of management is helpful—leadership concepts in particular. When you are in the midst of a health or life crisis, this kind of terminology may be far away from conscious thought, which is all the more reason to consider it now if you are less stressed, wary, or weary. You may find you need additional information and clarification of the whole management process and that you may be helped by more detailed information, more instruction, or more clarification. There are many books available—some that are free and some that are targeted to health care. Later, what you are learning or reviewing now can become subliminal, giving love and compassion more space and place.

For the remainder of this chapter, I'll explain these concepts with tie-ins to the story of my father inserted throughout. If you are already well-grounded in business or if you are so fatigued you may quit reading, then, by all means, just scan the management process information while focusing on the application tie-ins. But consider returning to it all at some later date.

To accomplish any goal, especially if it is providing care for someone you love, we all need a process of effectively and efficiently planning, organizing, leading, and controlling the activities of people and resources in achieving your purpose. We need to think about delineating objectives or expectations and realize they may be constantly changing and requiring periodic or continuous adjustment or fine-tuning. Those changing objectives are ours to decide, most likely such things as good medical decisions, comfort for all involved, opportunities for expressions of love and joy, and a sense of gratitude—some of which my own family made subordinate rather than paramount.

Motivating, staffing, coordinating, and communicating are additional things that will be in your management decision basket. Each of those management functions is of equal importance; all are needed. For effective outcomes, however, remember to coordinate, coordinate, coordinate.

Circumstances may determine sequencing the management functions as you cover the basics. Whoever takes on the job of managing must oversee both management activities and people. In our personal lives, we usually do not consider all the interactions of people, things, and processes that go into our decision choices, so we have given little thought to what may matter. With end-of-life care, whether your profession or your personal endeavor, it helps to have a sense of what needs overseeing, what matters, and what matters most.

Briefly, someone must monitor:

Planning: setting goals and determining the actions necessary to attain them; creating a course of action for achieving desired results/ objectives. Though planning is the usual starting point in managing, it may not feel that way when a medical emergency has occurred or an unexpected diagnosis has been given. You start from wherever you find yourself; you can make adjustments when needed. In the eighteenth century, Samuel Johnson cautioned, "Nothing will ever be attempted if all possible objections must first be overcome."

With my father, our early plan was to find a way to find out if recalibrating his prescriptions might make him more consistently comfortable. We saw only a single goal, used information from his current attending physicians, and acted thereon. In retrospect, that plan may have had seriously constraining parameters. We had limited ourselves. In our defense, we felt pushed by the obvious changes in Dad's well-being and, with limited information, started where we thought most pertinent. Sometimes you just do the best you can, and you continue through the process, improving as you go.

Organizing: bringing the resources (people, things, activities) together and using them in ways that help you get the outcomes you want. Organization is a process as well as it is a structure. It helps you determine the resources and activities required to achieve your goals. It can change as needs change. Be careful to pay more attention to the reasons for your organization than to your organizational structure itself. Keep your eye on outcomes so that you can change your organization to meet your goals. End-of-life care is not evenly paced or free of surprises.

For Dad's day-to-day in-home care, we had round-the-clock sitters who kept a journal of when and what he ate or drank, of his bodily eliminations, of the distribution of his medications, of his visitors, and of anything else they or we felt was significant. We consulted with them on our daily trips to his home, which we three siblings did separately at varying times. But with his physicians, we ceded to their judgment, prescriptions, and recommendations. Once we agreed to take him to the hospital, our organization was ceded and the goal kept limited. And the results were less than satisfactory. In hindsight, would we have done it differently? At the very least, I think we would have asked a lot more questions before making our decision.

Leading: using influence to motivate others to achieve your goals for your loved one and the family. You'll need to get others to do the things you need them to do, which may require giving guidance, instruction, and incentives. That involves your qualities, styles, and power, as well as effective communication, motivation, and discipline. Effective leadership really is a reciprocal process—two-way—and much of the time the interaction is face-to-face. Tasks are assigned, instructions given, feedback requested and supplied, and coaching provided if/when needed. And remember to be kind and polite to everyone, even when it is sometimes difficult to do. Especially with end-of-life care, courtesy, kindness, and consideration are big components of leading.

With Dad, we temporarily ceded our leadership to a psychiatrist who, by better balancing his medications, purportedly could help Dad respond more positively to his end-of-life changes and resulting anxieties. An internist was only modestly involved in our requests for additional insight and information. I did get in touch with a personal friend, another psychiatrist, hoping to find a way out of our dilemma. I failed, and we failed to see that we needed a more family-centered managerial approach on medical care, in addition to that of his in-home living care. Insufficient data gathering in planning and organizing, one might argue, negatively affected our later ability to lead or to influence the designated leader.

Controlling: a way of following up to ensure that your goals are being met. It helps you avoid doing the wrong things. Controlling is about establishing standards of performance, measuring work in progress, interpreting results, and making changes if required. Some treat control as the soul of the management process, because without planning, there is nothing to control, and without control, planning is a wasted exercise. Plans do not give positive results automatically; you'll consistently have to use control concepts to be sure you are getting the results you want. It is unwise to think mistakes can somehow be avoided; they can't. Be open and ready to modify your plans.

With our dad in the hospital, we had minuscule control. We had given that away for as long as he was there. In an attempt to wrestle some of it back, we made an appointment with the hospital social worker assigned to his case. She said she was sorry but that she was constrained by a physician's instructions—one who had said if our dad was released before his medications had been recalibrated, that he neither could nor would vouch for Dad's well-being. In hindsight, that seems the cruelest of jokes. Our dad was miserable, and so were we. I'm still not sure what we might have done differently, and there is no point in brutally castigating ourselves. It is pointless to place blame on ourselves or others. One suggestion for us all is to be as thorough as we can in learning what we need to know before the fact, not after. We will not achieve perfect knowledge, of course. Think it through as thoroughly as you can: what control will be available, and how much will you need? Even so, recognize that end-of-life care can bring rapid and unexpected changes. With Dad, we did not even consider we could be precipitating that possibility.

In our continuous vigilance, we also need to enhance effective management efforts by:

Motivating: inspiring and encouraging people to work with us, to take more interest and initiative in what is meaningful to the patient and family, to contribute more to achieving familial objectives for total care of all involved, for managing peripheral issues as well as medical ones. We all do better work and put forth more effort in a spirit of approval rather than one of criticism. Use positive strokes liberally and corrective ones cautiously.

A few motivational attempts come to mind—a seemingly

insignificant one in particular. The stress of admitting Dad to the psychiatric ward and the increasingly harsh restrictions on the family strained our relationships with some of his attending hospital personnel. I wanted to take an incentive—a love offering. Almost every week since my mother had died, as she had done, I baked a Bundt cake for Dad. He ate a small slice daily and shared it with his sitters and guests. *That's it,* I thought, and I baked one to take for the psych unit staff's break room, telling the on-duty nurses the cake story and encouraging them to take one small piece to Dad and share the rest. Yes, the intimate personal history of that small gesture helped a little to lighten our communication with them and to improve their cooperation with us.

Staffing: recruiting, selecting, appraising, and remunerating the right people. Staffing needs can shift and change as the needs of the loved one and family change. Choose carefully and consider that each one of the staff, new or continuing, will respond more to how much you care than how much you know. That is easy to forget in emotionally draining times.

Though the staffing at the hospital seemed beyond our control, perhaps it was not. I do remember talking only once to an officer of the hospital whom we knew, though not well, but he was reticent to be involved in medical care protocols—sympathetic, but of the-doctor-knows-best school of thought. Remember, our direct information became more limited as a physician restricted our visiting numbers and times. We can't change that past, but I have raised the question for you now.

Home caregiving required continuous monitoring. And changes were made. In one instance, we had to ask for skilled help. Eventually, one of our longest-employed caregivers, whom my father particularly liked, was convicted in a court of law of elder abuse. To collect the evidence for that and to convince Dad, we had professional help. The expense for gathering sufficient evidence was small compared to what we learned had been cumulatively stolen. Perhaps more damaging was the emotional loss for my dad when he learned of the caregiver's duplicitously sweet behavior.

We had to constantly evaluate the ability to take care of Dad as his needs increased. Often, this took care of itself when a caregiver felt the job had become too physically or emotionally taxing; several tearfully apologized for having to leave. Sometimes, they would recommend a replacement who was better suited; sometimes, we had to use professional personnel services. Whichever way, we required legal documentation such as Social Security verification, arrest records, references, and drug testing (for which we paid). Ask for professional guidance about what you need, as the laws do change.

We also found and enrolled Dad in an on-call nurse staffing organization so that we could get immediate professional help in case of an unexpected caregiver absence.

Coordinating: integrating activities of all persons—professional, family, and friends—who contribute to accomplishing your objectives. In business, some say this would be a part of organizational efforts. Because you have no formal organization and no business structure, you'll need to put a separate emphasis on coordination. Sometimes, this may be a bit frustrating, but it is hugely important. Remember, you'll not always please everyone.

With our dad, my brother, sister, and I had informal division of labor and responsibility. As he became less able to care for himself, we upped our participation. He was quite remarkable, actually, at saying without reticence, "I can't do this anymore." When he learned he had macular degeneration, he gave us his car keys; when he could no longer see well enough to sign his checks, he gave us the authority. Among us, we decided who would be primarily responsible for what, and we kept each other and Dad informed of everything.

For instance, one of us had Dad's power of attorney and took care of most business issues, only consulting the others on nonroutine matters, but informing the others about everything. Almost everything about house and home care were ceded to the other two, who found an informal way of dividing those decisions. But we all three kept each other informed of everything, as discussed below.

There were times we were not in agreement on the who, what, when, where, and in what ways, so we had to work at that. Yes, sometimes we were not all three equally satisfied with what we were doing. An illness doesn't stand still for unanimity of thinking, and so you will need to devise ways for cooperating without expecting perfection.

Communicating: a continuing process of telling, listening, and understanding, whether written or spoken; requires a constant exchange of facts, opinions, guidance, instructions, ideas, and information. If you listen to others, they are more apt to listen to you. Do the best you can to understand a situation before you make judgments about it. Ask questions when you need to know more.

Thank heavens for the internet. What an incredibly helpful tool for finding information we needed and for keeping each other constantly informed. In the last months, we siblings wrote to each other a lot, sending simultaneous emails. We could copy documents to share and forward information sent by health professionals, business persons, friends, or other family. In this way, we could also decide in what ways we wanted to reply to or to inform others and which of us would do that. Yes, we still talked on the phone (no texting at that time) and got together for discussions.

Especially with something that usually occurs around the edges of a basic management environment, someone assumes a leadership role—one of influencing others in establishing and realizing goals. As goals shift with situational changes, the leadership role within your caregiving team may also shift, whether family member or health-care professional. Whomever that is must be able to work effectively with others, to influence them toward mutually creating and fulfilling goals, and to bring about balance among individual and team goals. The successful leader gets others to follow. Kindness and caring are especially important for loving to the end … and on.

Within your team, who might be interacting with whom?

- medical staff and practitioners
- patient and medical personnel
- family members and medical personnel
- family members and significant others
- patient and family members and significant others
- support personnel such as religious leaders, sociologists, and nonmedical
- therapists with patient, family, and/or medical personnel
- all of the above with each other

As a team, you are more likely to work together in an atmosphere of trust and accountability toward shared goals. You'll put aside turf issues and politics to focus on what needs doing. A good decision-making process involves knowing what will be accepted and enthusiastically supported by your team of family, professionals, and supportive caregivers. Then, you are better positioned to use your loving resources to overcome barriers, to help identify new opportunities, and to develop momentum that leads to better problem-solving, more effective use of resources, and better outcomes.

Each of your team members needs to have commitment to an agreed common purpose. Each needs to stay involved until his or her role in an objective is completed. Often, this is subliminal when the team is functioning smoothly. That is best achieved when team members care about each other, including being concerned about how their actions and attitudes affect the patient and each other. Each needs to listen, respecting all points of view, and being sensitive to each other's needs. Each needs to be committed to keeping others informed. Though leadership, and even team composition, may shift while traveling to the end ... and on, each leader, when possible and appropriate, needs to encourage everyone's participation in the decisions to be made. As the end of life is increasingly near, leadership may shift more dramatically to family members; some medical personnel may need to be gently reminded. Team buy-in generally reinforces commitment. The love quotient for everyone is magnified.

Because Dad was the focus of us all, I can make a case for his having been the lead manager—the team leader. The values passed on to me and my siblings by our parents acted as unstated objectives: Act lovingly. Take care of each other. Be respectful. Remember, it's not over till it's over.

And it isn't over. It continues to the end ... and on.

Throughout, you can help yourself to understand yourself and your relationship to what is happening and to others in a fun, yet practical way. If you choose to learn more about yourself, you will also learn that the ways you interact, express, and present yourself can be linked to personal thinking, listening, and ways of communicating.

10

Listening to Yourself to Listen Better to Others

My eyes were drawn to the large, captioned lead story of the "Personal Journal" section of the *Wall Street Journal*: "How to Talk to Your Nurse,"[45] a piece written to and for health professionals, as well as patients and their families. Not surprisingly, you are reminded that communication between a patient's family and a nurse is vital and also vital with a physician. Patients and families are advised to ask questions, to be active participants in care, and to be unafraid to question actions you suspect are being made in error or may create a safety risk. Even so, you are cautioned to trust all medical personnel, especially the frontline nurses who work very hard, but then told you are the expert on your loved one. If you disagree with the care personnel, you are encouraged to approach the issue in a noncombative way. You may benefit from help with some ways to do that.

What needs doing during end-of-life care can strain even the most loving and giving of hearts, whether you are a family member or a part of a health-care team. As a loved one is increasingly dependent, caregivers lose some independence. So many things change, sometimes very rapidly, though sometimes slowly in a painfully prolonged way. It is no wonder that *The 36-Hour Day,* a book first published in 1981 by Nancy Mace, MA and Peter V. Rabins, MD, MPH, is in its fifth edition.

Besides learning all the external options you have with caregivers, caregiving facilities, helpful gadgets, and beneficial relaxation aids, there is something else you can do. Family caregiver or professional caregiver, you can learn more about your own personal thinking styles or preferences. The ways you think affect what you say, what you do, and how you do it. Your preferred thinking style affects how people respond to you and the ways in which they are willing to work with you. It affects your ability to get your needs met and the needs of your loved one accommodated.

There are times when end of life happens rapidly and unexpectedly. There are so many things that have to be done: Legal requirements to satisfy. Religious protocols to honor. Family traditions to follow. Thinking may feel blurred by fear, sorrow, or shock. The way you act, the things you do, and the way you communicate may be almost rote, coming from deep within, from your place of comfort, and from your most usual way of thinking.

In unexpected or in more normal circumstances, your unique manner of thinking propels the things you say, the way you say them, and the way you hear the answers. Fortunately, there is a practical path for exploring your preferred ways of thinking—one not requiring exploration of complex brain physiology. Once you get the basics, it's easier to either understand a situation or to change it, or maybe both. Why do this? You do this because you can, because you want to destress, and because you want to take the best possible care of your loved one, of those who help with your loved one, and of yourself. It isn't quite as simple as just thinking about your thinking. So fortunately, there is a tool that is helpful for glimpsing what your brain likes and what your brain-directed thinking preferences might be. Before describing that tool, I want to be clear that I use mind, brain, and thinking style terminology as metaphors for what really may be happening, whether from within our physical beings or from some source about which we continue to learn.

In the late 1970s, while he was working as manager of management education at General Electric's Management Development Institute, Ned Herrmann developed his Whole Brain® Model and Whole Brain Technology® metaphors for illustrating ways the brain works.[46]

His neuropsychological research used a physiological basis. That later shifted to a metaphorical model based on documentation of observable behaviors and the creation of the HBDI® Assessment, which gives you a really good way to learn about your personal thinking style. You don't need to remember any of that to be helped by what Ned created. (Whole Brain® is a registered trademark of Herrmann Global, LLC. Registered in the U.S. Patent and Trademark Office.)

The Herrmann Brain Dominance Instrument®[47] is like holding up a mirror so you can glimpse your thinking style preferences, the way your thinking works, its effects on your interactions, and the ways you can use knowing those things to help yourself and others. You'll figure out reasons some people understand you better than others and why you do the same. The HBDI®[48] simplifies the immensely complex activities of our thinking. Even so, thankfully, it provides insightful, useful information for helping you figure out what is going on in your environment, what may need to be done, and who might be the best suited to do so. With end-of-life care, it is also very useful in helping you find the helpers or team members you may need, when you may need different ones, ways you might shift duties or responsibilities around, and what else may need to happen.

So what does it do? The Herrmann Whole Brain® Model shows four distinct yet interconnected thinking styles, which metaphorically represents the specialized thinking modes that you access most frequently, organized into a four-quadrant model. Sounds more complicated than it is. Relax. (Whole Brain® is a registered trademark of Herrmann Global, LLC. Registered in the U.S. Patent and Trademark Office.)

For our purposes, we will highlight just a few of the ideas and revelations you will enjoy if you explore the HBDI® Profile[49] more fully. You'll have a few aha moments about yourself and about others with whom you work and for whom you are providing care.

Some people find it helpful to think of the four specialized modes of the Whole Brain® model in the form of selves you act out in response to everyday situations. The rational self, A quadrant: the analyzer enjoys processing numbers, analysis of facts, quantifying, being realistic, knowing about money, and understanding how things work. The safekeeping self, B quadrant: the organizer enjoys establishing procedures, planning approaches, taking preventive action, organizing facts, and making detailed reviews. The feeling self, C quadrant: the personalizer likes to teach, touch, and be supportive; is sensitive to others; and is interpersonal, emotional, expressive, and intuitive about others. The experimental self, D quadrant: the strategizer infers, speculates, and conceptualizes; is imaginative; is holistic and curious; is playful; takes risks; and will often break rules.[50] Little bits of each of the quadrant styles are needed for loving to the end ... and on.

To illustrate, let's assume a person has just been diagnosed with a malady of some kind. The A-quadrant oriented person might say something like, "I'd like a comparative analysis of probable treatment options, costs, and outcomes." The B-quadrant oriented person would ask for a list of each alternative treatment and its frequency of use, the time frame for using each, and treatment providers with their individual ratings if possible. The C-quadrant oriented person will want to know what will make the patient and the family the most comfortable physically, emotionally, and spiritually. And the D-quadrant oriented person will want to go beyond most-often used treatments in order to explore outside of traditional boundaries. And if there is nothing new, he might suggest using what exists to create something specifically for a patient, asking if anyone had thought outside the box. There is nothing wrong, of course, with any of those; they are just different in process and approach.

Each in this example is simplified, as the research shows we all have access to all four quadrants of the Whole Brain®[51] thinking model. And each might yield very different outcomes. Obviously, a team with persons who can collectively cover all of those possibilities is an excellent option to have. (Whole Brain® is a registered trademark of Herrmann Global, LLC. Registered in the U.S. Patent and Trademark Office.)

This does not mean that a team must have a minimum of four persons; there can be fewer, because any individual will typically have more than one preference—two, three, or even all four thinking preferences—that may be accessed more readily. Irrespective of the preferences, you can learn to shift your thinking to any quadrant and probably already do so! For taking care of yourself and loved ones needing care, just realizing in what way you are most likely to think about and assess things can remind you that there is something you may be missing. Then you can make choices about what else you may need to know or to do and whom you might approach for that help.

Thinking styles are not about intelligence, though they can have an effect on competence and results, depending on the nature of the task. I encourage you to spend a little time reflecting on yourself so that you can be more confident in your own decisions and in getting any kind of situational help you need from those whose thinking strengths will complement yours. Is there a quadrant (see preceding paragraph) you think describes you? Is there a quadrant where you think, *Me? Never!* If there is, in what ways do you find help for those tasks? Who helps?

When under stress, a prior understanding of thinking styles and how people process patient care activities can be hugely valuable. As you become increasingly aware of your HBDI®[52] thinking style preferences, you have a clearer perspective of yourself in relation to others. And you offer information in a way that recognizes, respects, and is compatible with different preferences for family members and friends or for coworkers, patients, and patient families' needs, hopes, and expectations. When you are able to recognize and appreciate differences, you increase your flexibility and effectiveness.[53] You will enjoy being understood, lessening your own frustrations, and satisfying coworkers, patients, or family.

The payoff for learning to recognize the traits in yourself and others is that you'll find it both easier to identify any assistance you need and to more confidently assist others. Your Whole Brain®[54] thinking style preferences are neither good nor bad, but knowing the ways to use them can be very, very good. (Whole Brain® is a registered trademark of Herrmann Global, LLC. Registered in the U.S. Patent and Trademark Office.)

If you are a professional caregiver, I strongly recommend you visit the website of Herrmann International®.[55] And I even more strongly recommend you invest in learning about your own HBDI® Profile in more detail.[56] Because you understand that we simply think differently, you'll be less apt to label other people or assign them a type, which is not an appropriate use of this model. When you make an effort to relate to the thinking preference of another, you will choose words or actions that are more comfortable for the other, becoming even more skilled getting done what needs doing.

Just one quick example may help. Do not expect, for example, a typical radiologist to rush to a family member's side and give a hug. Chances are, if one chooses radiology, one enjoys detailed analysis, looking at imaging of bodies rather than personally interacting with those bodies, or especially with the personalities therein—probably strong A and B quadrant (left mode) HBDI®[57] thinking preferences. Pediatricians differ from that markedly; many of their patients are preverbal and benefit most from caring touch and nonverbal communications—probably strong C and D (right mode) thinking preferences. These two examples are greatly simplified but give a sense of what you can learn, decreasing your frustration with wanting every caregiver to exhibit all possible behaviors with equal alacrity.

If you are a family member caregiving near the end of life for a loved one, I salute you if you have been able to read this chapter. If you have been able to grasp any of what it offers, that is wonderful. If not, just keep on loving. You are living a very stressful period of your life. When you assess or you sense that knowing more about this will be of service to you, you can proceed and profit from Ned Herrmann's work.

If you are a professional caregiver or medical practitioner, I encourage you to take a deeper look at ways you think and the related behaviors.[58] I remember once working with the lead twenty professionals in a psychiatric hospital in an effort to improve their teamwork. Each had completed the HBDI®[59] Profile. When I divided them into discussion groups organized by similar profile preferences, they were asked to discuss what they thought of the work and communications styles represented by each of the four quadrants. As expected, the primarily A-quadrant dominant officers, when asked about the work preferences of primarily D-quadrant officers, retorted, "They call that work?" And in reverse, I had expected that the primarily D-quadrant officers would reply the usual, "Boring." But not at this psychiatric hospital: with hilarity, they blurted out, "Anal retentive."

The point being, each HBDI®[60] thinking style has its strengths, and each has its weaknesses. You can benefit from sharing strengths, from ceding leadership in accordance to needs, and from developing good teamwork to maximize potential of a caregiver group, and that includes family members on whom professionals and their patients rely for many peripheral management decisions. You will find yourself less frustrated and more able to untangle or avoid messy personal interactions. There will be more time for loving to the end … and on.

(HBDI®, Whole Brain® and all related terms designated as ® are registered trademarks of Herrmann Global, LLC.)

11

Considering Impossibly Possible

There really is no explanation or prescription for loving and for being with and available to those you love until the last breath and then on. And there is no one way to provide the best possible care for your loved one or for yourself and others who are the caregivers.

In *Knocking on Heaven's Door, the Path to a Better Death,* Katy Butler tells the story of her father's painfully prolonged life, made by decisions she later questioned.[61] She explains the ways in which those decisions led her mother to reject medical recommendations for extending her own life. And as eye-opening as the narrative of her story is, even more so is Butler's chapter 20, "Notes for the New Art of Dying." She shares a personal exposé of what she learned the hard way and the options she uncovered. She offers herself and her parents to you as guides along usually dimly lit physical and emotional paths.

But what of the other, not physical aspects of life ending? If you have had difficulties with those parts of this book, please recall that in the beginning, you were asked to suspend your disbelief and to allow possibilities rather than automatically reject them. There is more you can do.

As you explore your perspective of reality, you may go beyond Newtonian materialism, which was probably the science you studied most in school. Without becoming a quantum physicist, you can venture forward into new learning—not a simple task. Superstring theory, exploring linkages among gravity and ten or more dimensions, and an eleventh dimensional M-theory of nondetectable energy fields exist mathematically and challenge the facts most of us learned about living in a three-dimensional universe. Ongoing exploration yields more and more theoretical constructs in search of answers to our deepest questions of how our universe began and the reasons behind the form we see on earth and in the heavens. As a nonscientist, I cannot claim to understand all of that, but my search continues for answers to universal questions.

Recently, scientists captured on film the fireworks of life beginning; there is a bright flash of light as a sperm meets an egg—an explosion of tiny sparks erupting from the egg at the moment of conception. And the research predicts that those eggs that burn brighter than others are more likely to produce a healthy baby.[62] Unrelated to the specific cause of death, there is also a death flash; it is independent of the cause of death and may reflect both the intensity and rate of dying.[63] Might there be information in the electromagnetic field that comes from necrotic radiation and in its energy, its information, that opens the possibility of consciousness beyond the body? I don't know; I am hoping to learn more.

When considering NDEs, for example, the experiencers describe what occurs during a period of clinical death. The numbers of reports and the studies of large numbers of NDEs across cultures and time present genuine evidence toward concluding that consciousness survives death. Or is it, perhaps, that we have failed to appropriately define consciousness or death or life or any combination thereof?[64]

For me, the personal stories that people of all walks of life and of all levels of education have shared are even more compelling. Sometimes these are secrets they've never shared with anyone else, often fearing they would be ridiculed or disbelieved, and so the joy of the experience would be tainted, lessened, or spoiled in some way.

In the early 1950s, several prominent singers recorded a love song for teens, "They Try to Tell Us We're Too Young." Nat King Cole took it to number one on the charts. Wanda and Justin were among the many high school students who thought of themselves as the couple in that song. They were like so many other young lovers who separated when families moved or college choices separated them.

But their hearts never truly separated. Decades and divorces later, including children with other spouses, Wanda and Justin married. As in the song, they recalled not having been too young at all.

After twenty-one years of marriage, Justin's health deteriorated rapidly. His death was devastating for Wanda. In the early weeks and months after he died, she spent a lot of time traveling to be with other family members. During one cold trip to Utah ski territory, at night Wanda and some of her family stood in a sheltered area watching skiers coming down star-lit slopes. A light snow began to fall—magically beautiful. Telling me about it, Wanda said, "Lynn, I can tell you this, because you'll understand. A snowflake fell, hitting my lip, and I knew it was a kiss from Justin. I just knew." She spoke through tears. Hers is another example of loving beyond death. I think of it as the snowflake that was a kiss. When we are open, the impossibly possible does happen.

A few days after her husband's funeral, Betty had come to visit with me in my home. She knew that sometimes I'd been able to intuit messages from others, both living and no longer in physical bodies. She hoped, maybe, in some way I might help her with her grief. I hurt to see how deeply she was grieving. Because something worn by another person sometimes has acted like an information conduit for me, I asked to hold something of Jason's. She handed me his gold wedding ring. While holding it, I mentioned several different things I sensed, but nothing seemed to get Betty's attention until I mentioned shoes and then added that Jason wanted to thank her for the wonderfully comfortable slippers. Betty wrinkled her brow and cocked her head a bit but couldn't bring forward any specifically meaningful memory—that is, until she returned from Alabama to their apartment in Chicago. At home, she opened the downstairs closet door and saw the warm, really lovely, shearling-lined leather slippers she had bought for him the previous winter, having chosen them for comfort and ease of taking them on and off, which had been a big help as Jason's balance had become troubling. Those were the only shoes in the downstairs coat closet, with boots being left in the garage and other shoes in the bedroom. Betty looked again at the slippers, closed the closet door, and worked at various tasks throughout the day, with periodic wonderings about those slippers. Night came, and on her way to bed, Betty walked by that closet.

Its door was wide open; she closed it, leaving the slippers there. For weeks, this became routine. The door would be open, and she would close it. Then she'd find it open again. Betty was amused and comforted by the feeling that Jason was there every time the door was open. "It wasn't just a mild feeling about Jason's presence," Betty explained to me. "It felt like the door was deliberately being left opened, and Jason's presence was very real."

Jason and Betty are both PhD chemists, noted researchers, university professors, and patent holders. More than a week after Jason died, choosing to avoid her coworkers, Betty started going to her office at work either early in the morning or in the evening. Jason's office was to the south and one over from hers. All of the offices on their wing faced east and looked out over the lagoon. Because the windows are coated to keep heat in during winter, they look semireflective inside when it's dark outside.

About one week after Jason's death, an especially nice and talented PhD student stopped by to tell Betty how shocked and sad he was about her husband's death, saying it had been just hours earlier when another grad student told him about Jason's dying. Describing the reason for his surprise, he explained, "I was sitting at my desk a couple of nights ago facing the windows, my back to the door, and I saw your husband walking by, his reflection in the window. So, I said, 'Hi, Dr. J,' and he waved back at me." That greeting was days after his death. Jason had also really liked and appreciated this student, a Christian from Eritrea.

Sharing with me that she often enjoyed talking to the Eritrean, as well as a couple of Ethiopian Christian grad students about their lives, culture, and faith, Betty has commented that each of them seemed very much in tune with the supernatural and mystical. How wonderful that her openness and interest had allowed their sharing a hallowed experience.

There are also sacred moments before death. Carrie and I had been friends since preschool. As ALS began to limit her movements, I would sometimes put both her wheelchair and walker into my trunk, so we'd be prepared for whichever she'd need when we'd take off, laughing continuously, for an undecided location for lunch or whatever we might decide. As her moving and breathing became more taxing, we were limited to in-home visits. With her condition worsening, the pragmatic businesswoman also began discussing end-of-life options with her physician, including her preference for hospice care. Eventually, when sniffles became pneumonia, she was hospitalized.

A few days later, at around six o'clock, during early morning rounds, her physician came to her room. Knowing death was imminent, "she told him that she was ready for the hospice care they had already discussed. I was caught off guard," her daughter Audrey said, "when she told him that she was ready on that day, or maybe it was just the shock of hearing her give up, of knowing death was near. She fought so hard for so long, and I don't think any of us knew how great her struggle was, every hour of every single day."

The attending physician agreed and said he would make arrangements immediately, explaining again for Carrie and for Audrey how hospice pain management would work.

Seeing her daughter's tears, Carrie said, "Please don't cry, honey. I'm just so tired, and I can't fight it anymore." She knew that hospice could help to modify her sometimes-severe discomfort through the use of drugs, that the relaxation provided by those drugs might inhibit her already-compromised speech, and that she would rest better and sleep more and more deeply.

With the decision made, Audrey said, "I called Cindy [her sister] so she could hurry down and then called you."

My clock showed a little before seven o'clock in the morning when the phone rang. After I said hello, I heard, "Lynn, this is Audrey. Momma said you're an early riser, and she wants to talk to you."

Then I heard Carrie, her voice wispy and soft. "Hospice help will be here soon, so I want to tell you now. I love you."

Just as I said the same back to her, Audrey's voice again. "We've got to go now. The hospice nurse is here with pain medication. You can tell some of the others."

The others were additional childhood friends. The plan had been for Carrie to call several of us, but that wasn't to happen. "She wanted so badly to call everyone," Audrey explained later, "but she just didn't have enough breath."

I am forever grateful to be the early riser.

Though our conscious extension of love is a continuing sacred gift, it does not mean that I am okay with having my friend less accessible. What is apparent to me is the strength of physical interaction. I am always aware in talking to people about loving beyond death how much the physical misses the physical: the sound of a voice, the feel of skin touching skin, the smell of a favorite perfume or aftershave, the taste of one's lips on another, and the shared laughter or tears. Though it is true that some of us are, from my point of view, blessed with the ability to receive a physical sensation from someone no longer in a physical body, it is usually fleeting and rarely on command. Even a brief interaction, however, gives promise of existence beyond our physical limits.

As Hugh reminded me, *"Love is indestructible."* To gain a deeper understanding of death or the dying process, then, we needn't prove or disprove an afterlife—a consciousness that survives death. But we can explore and open our hearts and minds, and in doing so, dying patients' care may be enhanced. Our own lives may be magnified. Perhaps, we need only to become vulnerable, simply loving those who are leaving, wherever they are, however they may be experiencing reality as it is revealed to them. And in doing that, we may confront our own limitations while expanding our options. We will choose to love openly, freely, and with the possibility—for me, the probability—that we can, indeed, enjoy loving fully to the end … and on.

Writing in the nineteenth century, Henry Ward Beecher noted, "Love is the river of life in this world." Or is it, perhaps, that love is the river that flows into, throughout, and beyond life in this physical world?

Resources: A Beginning Few

Books:

General

Arcangel, Dianne and Gary Schwartz. *Afterlife Encounters: Ordinary People, Extraordinary Experiences.* Charlottesville, VA: Hampton Roads Publishing Co., 2005.

Bell, Carmel. *When All Else Fails: A Journey into the Heart with Medical Intuition and Metatronic Energy*. Brisbane, Australia: Book Pal, 2010.

Betty, Stafford. *When Did You Ever Become Less by Dying? AFTERLIFE: The Evidence.* Guildford, Surrey United Kingdom: White Crow Books, 2016.

Bulkeley, Kelly, and Rev. Patricia Bulkeley. *Dreaming Beyond Death: A Guide to Pre-Death Dreams and Visions*. Boston, MA: Beacon Press, 2005.

Burke, John. *Imagine Heaven: Near-Death Experiences, God's Promises, and the Exhilarating Future That Awaits You*. Grand Rapids, MI: Baker Books, 2015.

Butler, Katy. *Knocking on Heaven's Door: The Path to a Better Way of Death*. New York: Scribner, 2013.

Clark, Nancy. *Stop Trying to Fix Me: I'm Grieving* as *Fast as I Can.* Fairfield, IA: 1st World Publishing, 2013.

Coward, Harold. *Life after Death in World Religions (Faith Meets Faith).* Maryknoll, NY: Orbis Books, 1997.

Geiger, John. *The Third Man Factor: Surviving the Impossible.* New York: Weinstein Books, 2009.

Hemingway, Annamaria. *Practicing Conscious Living and Dying: Stories of Eternal Continuum or Consciousness.* Ropley, Hants, UK: O Books, John Hunt Publishing,, 2008.

Huguenot, Alan Ross. *The Death Experience: What It Is Like When You Die.* Indianapolis, IN: Dog Ear Publishing, 2012.

Humphrey, Derek. *Final Exit: The Practicalities of Self-Deliverance and Assisted Suicide of the Dying,* Third Edition, New York: Dell Publishing, 2002.

Johnson, Christopher Jay and Marsha G. McGee, eds. *How Different Religions View Death & Afterlife.* Philadelphia, PA: Charles Press Publishers, 1998.

Jovanovic, Pierre. *An Inquiry into the Existence of Guardian Angels: A Journalist's Investigative Report.* English translation. New York: M. Evans and Company, 1995.

Kelly, E.F., E.W. Kelly, A. Crabtree, A. Gauld, M. Grosso, and B. Greyson. *Irreducible Mind: Toward a Psychology for the 21st Century.* Lanham,Maryland: Rowman and Littlefield Publishers, Inc., 2007.

Kessler, David. *The Needs of the Dying: A Guide for Bringing Hope, Comfort, and Love to Life's Final Chapter.* New York: Quill, 1997.

Larson, Cynthia Sue. *Reality Shifts: When Consciousness Changes the Physical World.* Berkeley, CA: Reality Shifters, 1999.

Mendoza, Marilyn A. *We Do Not Die Alone: "Jesus Is Coming to Get Me in a White Pickup Truck."* Dahlonega, GA: ICAN Publishing, 2009.

Mitchell, Edgar D. *Psychic Exploration: A Challenge for Science.* New York: G.P. Putnam's, 1974.

North, Carolyn. *The Experience of a Lifetime: Living Fully Dying Consciously*. San Francisco: Amber Lotus, 1998.

Rivas, Titus, Anny Dirven, and Rudolf H. Smit. *The* Self *Does Not Die: Verified Paranormal Phenomena from Near-Death Experiences*. Durham: NC: IANDS Publications, 2016.

Ruter Springer, Rebecca. *My Dream of Heaven*. Tulsa, OK: Harrison House Publishers, 1898.

Sharp, Kimberly Clark. *After the Light: What I Discovered on the Other Side of Life That Can Change Your World*. New York: William Morrow and Co., 1995.

Steiger, Brad, and Sherry Hansen Steiger. *Miracles of Healing: Inspirational Stories of Amazing Recovery*. Avon, MA: Adams Media, 2004.

Sudman, Natalie. *Application of Impossible Things: My Near Death Experience in Iraq*. Huntsville, AR: Ozark Mountain Publishing, 2012.

Tremblay, Robert M. *Twenty-Seconds: A True Account of Survival & Hope*. Bloomington, IN: Balboa Press, 2015.

Wilcock, David. *The Synchronicity Key*. New York: Dutton, 2013.

Written by Physicians

Bellg, Laurin. *Near Death in the ICU: Stories from Patients Near Death and Why We Should Listen to Them*. I: Sloan Press, 2016.

Charbonier, Jean Jacques. *7 Reasons to Believe in the Afterlife: A Doctor Reviews the Case for Consciousness After Death*. Rochester, VT: Inner Traditions, 2015.

Gawande, Atul. *Being Mortal, Medicine, and What Matters in the End*. New York: Metropolitan Books, 2014.

Hamilton, Allan J. *The Scalpel and the Soul: Encounters with Surgery, the Supernatural, and the Healing POWER OF HOPE*. New York: Jeremy P. Tarcher/Penguin, 2008.

Kircher, Pamela M. *Love Is the Link: A Hospice Doctor Shares Her Experience of Near-Death and Dying* Burdett, NY: Larson Publications, 1995.

Kübler-Ross, Elizabeth. *On Death and Dying: What the Dying Have to Teach Doctors, Nurses, Clergy, and Their Own Families.* New York: Macmillan Publishing Co., 1969.

———. *On Life After Death.* Berkeley, CA: Celestial Arts, 1991.

McCullough, Dennis. *My Mother, Your Mother: Embracing "Slow Medicine," the Compassionate Approach to Caring for Your Aging Loved Ones.* New York: Harper Collins, 2009.

Moody, Raymond A., Jr. *Life After Life.* New York: Bantam, 1975.

———. *Reunions: Visionary Encounters with Departed Loved Ones.* New York Villard Books, 1993.

Moody, Raymond A., Jr. with Paul Perry. *Coming Back: A Psychiatrist Explores Past-Life Journeys.* New York: Bantam Books, 1990.

———. *Glimpses of Eternity: Sharing of a Loved One's Passage from This Life to the Next.* New York: Guideposts, 2010.

———. *Paranormal, My Life in Pursuit of the Afterlife.* New York: Harper Collins, 2012.

Moody, Raymond, Jr., and Dianne Arcangel. *Life After Loss: Conquering Grief and Finding Hope.* New York: Harper San Francisco, 2001.

Morse, Melvin, with Paul Perry. *Parting Visions: Uses and Meanings of Pre-Death, Psychic, and Spiritual Experiences.* New York: Villard Books, 1994.

Neal, Mary. *To Heaven and Back: A Doctor's Extraordinary Account of Her Death, Heaven, Angels, and Life Again: A True Story.* Colorado Springs, CO: WaterBrook Press, 2011, 2012.

———. *7 Lessons from Heaven: How Dying Taught Me to Live a Joy-Filled Life.* New York: Convergent, 2017.

Newberg, Andrew, and Mark Robert Waldman. *How God Changes Your Brain: Breakthrough Findings from a Leading Neuroscientist*. New York: Ballantine Books, 2009.

Ritchie, George G., Jr. *Ordered to Return: My Life After Dying* Charlottesville, VA: Hampton Roads Publishing Co., 1998.

Sabom, Michael. *Light and Death*. Grand Rapids, MI: Zondervan Publishing House, 1998.

Sharkey, Frances. *A Parting Gift: A Profound and Moving Story*. New York: Bantam Books, 1982.

,t. *Our Life after Death: A Firsthand Account from an 18th-Century Scientist and Seer*. West Chester, PA: Swedenborg Foundation, 2014.

Vieira, Waldo. *Projections of the Consciousness: A Diary of Out-of-Body Experiences.*,Rio De Janeiro, RJ, Brazil: IIPC, 1997.

Whitton, Joel L., and Joe Fisher. *Life Between Life*. NYC:Warner Books, 1986.

Wyatt, Karen M. *What Really Matters: 7 Lessons for the Living from the Stories of the Dying*. Silverthorne, CO: Sunroom Studios, 2011.

Written by Nurses

Callanan, Maggie, and Patricia Kelley. *Final Gifts*. New York: Bantam Book, 1992.

Corcoran, Diane. *When Ego Dies: A Compilation of Near-Death & Mystical Conversion Experiences*. Houston, TX: Emerald Ink Publishing, 1996.

Karnes, Barbara. *The Final Act of Living: Reflections of a Longtime Hospice Nurse*. Depoe Bay, OR: Barbara Karnes Books, Inc., 2003.

Sartori, Penny. *The Wisdom of Near-Death Experiences: How Understanding NDEs Can Help Us Live More Fully*. New York: Osprey Publishing, 2014.

Wehr, Janet. *Peaceful Passages: A Nurse's Stories of Dying Well*. Wheaton, IL: Quest Books, 2015.

Science in General, Physics

Bray, William Joseph. *Quantum Physics, Near Death Experiences, Eternal Consciousness, Religion, and the Human Soul*. San Bernadino, CA: CreateSpace Independent Publishing Platform, 2012.

Greene, Brian. *The Elegant Universe: Superstrings, Hidden Dimensions, and the Quest of the Ultimate Theory*. New York: Norton & Co., 1999.

Pruett, Dave. *Reason and Wonder: A Copernican Revolution in Science and Spirit*. Santa Barbara, CA: ABC-CLIO, LLC, 2012.

Swanson, Claude. *Life Force, The Scientific Basis: Breakthrough Physics of Energy Medicine, Healing, Chi and Quantum Consciousness (Volume Two of the Synchronized Universe Series)*. Tucson, AZ: Poseidia Press, 2010.

Tart, Charles T. *The End of Materialism: How Evidence of the Paranormal Is Bringing Science and Spirit Together*. Oakland, CA: New Harbinger Publications, Inc., 2009.

Management and Management Related

Drucker, Peter F. *The Effective Executive: The Definitive Guide to Getting the Right Things Done*. New York: Harper Collins, 2006.

Herrmann, Ned. *The Creative Brain*. Lake Lure, NC: Brain Books, 1991.

———. *The Whole Brain Business Book: Unlocking the Power of Whole Brain Thinking in Organizations and Individuals*. New York: McGraw Hill, 1996.

Mosley,D.C. and Pietri,P.H.. *Supervisory Management: The Art of Inspiring, Empowering, and Developing People*. Stamford, CT: Cengage Learning, 2015.

Movies

There are many movies available to entertain you while reinforcing numerous particulars of end-of-life activities. It is important to remember, though, that movies are just that—entertainment. Some are more factually accurate than others, and you will need to be discerning in your use of what they represent. I shall list only a few that I recommend.

In the 1980 movie *Resurrection*, Ellen Burstyn plays Edna McCauley, the wife of a man who is killed in an auto crash. Edna survives, though it seems she has had an NDE, an OBE, or both. While recuperating, Edna discovers she is able to heal people, a possible byproduct of an NDE. As she struggles to understand near-death aftereffects, her life is changed completely. It was nominated for two Academy Awards.

In the 1984 movie *Dreamscape*, a physician who hopes to alleviate the pain of patients with recurring nightmares uses elements of ESP for exploration into the subconscious of patients. With an American president as one of the patients, the movie becomes somewhat of a thriller. Nonetheless, it raises important questions of the nature of consciousness.

The 1987 movie *Made in Heaven* is a fun, offbeat romance that includes accidental death, a trip to heaven where a deceased aunt explains the rules, encountering love in heaven, and an unexpected return to Earth with additional twists and turns. Though full of folly, its elements may enlarge your interest and analysis of what NDErs report. You may expand the questions you want to ask.

An incredibly popular film in 1990, *Ghost* takes after-death communication to new heights of hilarity and of drama. It mixes together comedy, romance, action, and yuckiness. There is both exaggeration and realism if you can discern the difference. *Ghost* was a huge hit and had five Academy Award nominations.

Because many NDErs report changes in their energy fields, in their capacities to do unusual things, and in a need to help others in whatever way they are able, the 1999 movie *The Green Mile* invites serious thought about illness, healing, and things unknown. Certainly, faith healers, shamans, and curanderos are different in beliefs, approach, and technique than Western medical practitioners.

This movie uses visual imagery to raise a question of the healing power of gentle love. It was nominated for four Academy Awards.

Few can forget the line in the 1999 movie *The Sixth Sense* when nine-year-old Cole whispers, "I see dead people." For those of us who are comfortable with after-death communication, it was a delight, even in the tenser moments. It was nominated for six Academy Awards.

The 2001 movie *Defending Your Life* has a star-studded cast whose characters find themselves doing life reviews in afterlife settings. Love, even romance, are engaging aspects of this philosophical comedy.

The 2002 film *Dragonfly* is a heart-wringing thriller. The plot involves use of information a physician learns through both the near-death experiences of his patients and after-death communication with his deceased wife. Its strong Hollywood cast keeps you engaged until its surprising conclusion.

The 2005 movie *Just Like Heaven* is a delightful romantic comedy with A-list Hollywood stars. A young emergency physician whose work has been her life exhibits aspects of NDE and OBE. A man grieving the sudden death of his wife becomes entwined with the physician's very active out-of-body experiences. There are many hospital scenes, including a miraculous recovery from coma.

The 2009 film version of the award-winning and best-selling 2002 novel *The Lovely Bones* tells the story of a viciously murdered fourteen-year-old girl who struggles to find footing in the hereafter where she meets other victims of her assailant and where she finds a way to briefly reenter the earth realm and move the plot toward its conclusion. Its afterlife story aspects are akin to some NDErs' comments.

In 2009 *The Men Who Stare at Goats* brought the story of remote viewing, as used by the military, to the big screen. Though the movie, in my opinion, does not do justice to the extraordinary skills or the science behind those skills that allow a person to give details about a target place or person that is inaccessible in distance or time to the normal senses, it is, at least, an introduction to remarkable abilities that can and are used in medicine too. Participants in military remote viewing, some key people at the Monroe Institute (see elsewhere in this book) have participated in serious and seriously studied remote viewing activity; many interviews with Joseph McMoneagle are available on YouTube. If you want to experience remote viewing for yourself, Paul H. Smith, PhD, retired military officer, offers learning possibilities: http://rviewer.com.

In 2014 Gayle Forman's best-selling (teen) novel came to the screen: *If I Stay*. Mia thought her decisions would be about pursuing her musical dreams at Julliard, but everything changed in an instant. This movie can now be found and viewed online for free.

In 2014 a best-selling book of the same name came to the screen: *Heaven Is for Real*. A small-town father struggles both with his son's insistence that during an NDE, he visited heaven and his son's matter-of-fact comments about things that happened before he had been born.

A 2015 Sundance prize winner, *Me and Earl and the Dying Girl*, is happy, funny, sad, and real in its portrayal of high school students who tell the story of friendship and terminal cancer. It illustrates the fun that is possible mixed with the pain that is often inevitable while loving to the end … and on.

A 2015 film, *The Farewell Party* (English subtitles), is the story of a group of friends in a Jerusalem retirement home. With humor, it tackles the difficult issues of aging, coping with pain, infirmity, and assisted suicide.

The 2015 film *One Cut, One Life* portrays the diagnosis and terminal illness of documentarian filmmaker Ed Pincus. He and his collaborator, Lucia Small, who also explores her feelings about the murders of two friends, make this one last film together. They invite you into the often intense, sometimes raw, and occasionally humorous exploration of end-of-life complexities. It is as much reflection as action in its format.

A 2016 movie based on a 2015 book, *Miracles from Heaven*, is a faith-based movie of parents dealing with an increasingly traumatic search for a cure for their ten-year-old daughter's usually incurable, rare disease. After the daughter has a freak accident, an extraordinary healing occurs, which the daughter reveals she was promised during a near-death experience.

Documentary Films

In 1975, Raymond A. Moody, Jr., MD, PhD, wrote *Life After Life: The Investigation of a Phenomenon—Survival of Bodily Death.* Dr. Moody is credited with creating the term NDE: near-death experience. In 1992 in a documentary-style production, Dr. Moody interviewed a diverse group of experiencers, including a Soviet dissident, a nurse, and others who are quite believable as they describe their experiences. Dr. Moody's dialogue throughout is entertaining and informative. And, if you are an internet user, it is available for you to view for free at: http://topdocumentaryfilms.com/life-after-life/.

In 1996, Dr. Elisabeth Kübler-Ross endorsed the documentary *Round Trip: The Near Death Experience.* Five people who have survived near-death experiences are interviewed: one whose body quit after eight years of debilitating illness, one who ran out of oxygen while scuba diving, one who had serious complications during childbirth, one who was tossed to the pavement when her tour bus flipped over, and one whose heart fluttered, then stopped, during surgery. Each of them left their bodies. A parapsychologist, a theologian, and a philosopher offer comments on these remarkably similar events. The film can be purchased at Amazon.com.

Training Video

The 2013 NDE training video *Near-Death Experience: What Medical Professionals Need to Know* may be ordered online at www.iands.org/video. The video features six medical professionals and a number of near-death experiences. It provides information and procedures to address the needs of patients who have had NDEs. It is also of interest to general audiences.

In the video, Dr. Laurin Bellg, critical care physician, entreats, "One of my hopes is that we can raise awareness among providers about the fact that this phenomenon does exist; whether it's something that we can prove scientifically or not actually becomes quite irrelevant. It is a subjective experience that the patient has that we need to honor and provide an invitation for patients to process that."

A trailer based on the video may be watched online at:

https://www.youtube.com/watch?v=ZxdNd5NnG1w&feature=youtu.be.

A DVD copy can also be ordered online at:

http://iands.org/resources/media-resources/front-page-news/969-nde-training-video-on-sale-september-10.html.

The NDE Medical Training Video comes in two forms:

- The thirty-minute DVD for near-death experiencers and general audiences
- The Training Package for hospitals, hospice, medical schools and nursing programs, which included the DVD plus:
    - o PowerPoint presentation
    - o Discussion questions
    - o Role play
    - o Reading lists
    - o Brochures for caregivers and experiencers
    - o And other training materials

Internet

With whatever search engine you prefer, you can find more than you will have time to pursue on the subjects in this book. Below you can choose among a wide variety of options that I have found helpful for my research, work, and personal use.

Incredibly helpful music: http://www.hemi-sync.com

I recommend the following, although there are numerous options for your choosing:

- Two-album set, valuable for anyone with a life-threatening condition and for the terminally ill and caregivers: Going Home series package with Hemi-Sync®
- Album series with six exercises for achieving the out-of-body state: Hemi-Sync® Support for Journeys Out of the Body
- Individual albums for rest and relaxation:Lullaby with Hemi-Sync® and Sleeping Through the Rain with Hemi-Sync®
- Cancer Support Series with Hemi-Sync®

Incredibly helpful guided imagery:

Belleruth Naparstek is the creator of Health Journeys acclaimed guided imagery audio series, with help for many specific physical and emotional difficulties. It can be found online at: http://www.healthjourneys.com.

Free guidebooks:

Brayne, Sue, and Peter Fenwick. *End-of-Life Experiences: A Guide for Carers of the Dying.* Braynework, 2008. (http://www.newcosmicparadigm.org/images/pdf/ENDOFLIFEPROF.pdf).

———. *Nearing the End of Life: A Guide for Relatives and Friends of the Dying.* In association with the Clinical Neuroscience Division University of Southampton (https://suebrayne.files.wordpress.com/2011/01/brochure.pdf).

Free management books:

http://bookboon.com/en/management-organisation-ebooks
(Bookboon is headquartered in the UK and Denmark with offices in Germany, Lithuania, the Netherlands, South Africa, Sweden and the USA.)

Peter Drucker, PhD:
http://www.druckerinstitute.com/peter-druckers-life-and-legacy/a-drucker-sampler/
http://druckerinst.dreamhosters.com/peter-druckers-life-and-legacy/

How to Talk to Your Doctor (or Any Member of Your Health Care Team):
http://theconversationproject.org/wp-content/uploads/2013/01/TCP-TalkToYourDoctor.pdf

Hospice worker experiences:

"Deathbed Visions: Hospice Nurses Share Their Stories"
https://www.youtube.com/watch?v=nMr_sapd-qY

Debunking Hospice Myths:

"Common Myths of Hospice Care Debunked"
http://www.forbes.com/sites/nextavenue/2015/02/25/common-myths-of-hospice-care-debunked/#44ed4a106973

Children related:

"Talking to Children about Death"
http://www.hospicenet.org/html/talking.html

"Children's Near-Death Experiences"
https://iands.org/childrens-near-death-experiences.html

"How School Counselors Can Assist Student Near-Death Experiencers"
http://www.biomedsearch.com/article/How-school-counselors-can-assist/245254049.html

Considering paths for end-of-life care:

Informational interview with Katy Butler on end-of-life care choices: http://www.c-span.org/video/?313011-9/book-discussion-knocking-heavens-door

Aftereffects of an NDE:

"Aftereffects of Near-Death States"
Written in 1998 and still appropriate, although more can be found online at: http://iands.org/aftereffects-of-near-death-states.html.

Religious beliefs and expectations for end of life:

"Customs and Religious Protocols: Different Cultural Beliefs at Time of Death"
http://amemorytree.co.nz/customs.php

"The Heart's Intuitive Intelligence"
https://www.heartmath.org/about-us/videos/the-hearts-intuitive-intelligence/

"Glimpses into the Afterlife"
http://www.reformjudaism.org/glimpses-afterlife

Personal stress-relief help for health professionals:

"Biofeedback Intervention for Stress and Anxiety among Nursing Students: A Randomized Controlled Trial"
https://www.heartmath.org/research/research-library/educational/biofeedback-intervention-for-stress-and-anxiety-among-nursing-students-a-randomized-controlled-trial/

A philosophical approach to death:

"Facing Death"
https://www.youtube.com/watch?v=oKSNhUDbmpE
Full lecture from Ram Dass in 1992. If an hour-plus video is unappealing, begin listening at about fifty minutes into the presentation and listen to the end.

Science and the Near-Death Experience:

"Science and the Near-Death Experience"
http://www.near-death.com/science/research/science.html

"Measurements on the Reality of the Wavefunction," Cornell University Library. Martin Ringbauer, Ben Duffus, Cyril Branciard, Eric G. Cavalcanti, Andrew G. White, Alessandro Fedrizzi (Submitted on December 19, 2014 (v. 1), last revised January 20, 2015 (this version, v. 2))

"Continuity of Consciousness," Pim van Lommel, MD
http://www.iands.org/research/important-research-articles/43-dr-pim-van-lommel-md-continuity-of-consciousness.html

"Science and Spirituality," Peter Fenwick, MD, FRCPsych
http://www.iands.org/research/important-research-articles/42-dr-peter-fenwick-md-science-and-spirituality.html

Physicians' experiences:

"Famous Cardiac Surgeon's Stories of Near Death Experiences in Surgery" (an interview with Dr. Lloyd Rudy)
https://www.youtube.com/watch?v=JL1oDuvQR08

"From Life to Death, Beyond and Back"
https://www.youtube.com/watch?v=mMYhgTgE6MU

Famous persons and near-death experiences:

"Celebrity Near-Death Experiences"
http://the-formula.org/celebrity-near-death-experiences/

Stories of life, death, and faith:

"To Heaven and Back" (Dr. Mary Neal, drowning; Anita Moorjani, cancer; Benjamin Breedlove, HCM)
http://www.cnn.com/2013/11/29/us/to-heaven-and-back/

Paul Kalanithi, MD, wrote essays for the *New York Times* and Stanford Medicine reflecting on being a physician and a patient, the human experience of facing death, and the joy he found despite terminal illness.
http://med.stanford.edu/news/all-news/2015/03/stanford-neurosurgeon-writer-paul-kalanithi-dies-at-37.html

Delving deeper:

"Edgar Mitchell"
http://noetic.org/directory/person/edgar-mitchell/

"Engineering and Consciousness"
http://www.princeton.edu/~pear/

"EKR Biography"
http://www.ekrfoundation.org/bio/elisabeth-kubler-ross-biography/

"Robert Monroe"
https://www.monroeinstitute.org/about/robert-monroe

Gratitude

In writing this book about loving to the end ... and on, I especially must acknowledge the generosity of love I have been given by

my husband and our two children, their spouses, and their children
my parents and their parents
my brother and sister, their spouses, and their children
my close cousins, their spouses, and their children
my childhood friends who remain so today, some still in bodies, some not, and their children

I have also been fortunate to make many more friends along the way who have generously loved me—business colleagues who have loved me and brief acquaintances who have reached out in love to me.

The friends made through the Intuition Network and through Inpresence have been an inspiration. Their experiences and their support have been long-lived and boundless.

I would specifically like to thank all of those who have assisted me in what became a more arduous task than I anticipated. Friends, family, and specifically Lourana Howard read, edited, and edited some more. The team of folks at Balboa Press who shepherded publication. Sara Sgarslat and her husband, Leonard, were invaluable help in getting information about this book to readers.

Ann Herrmann-Nehdi and her staff at Herrmann International were hugely supportive and helpful. Members and staff of the

International Association of Near-Death Studies provided help and support. Monroe Institute staff and fellow professional members provided inspiration. I am grateful to them all.

A special thanks to my friend who started this all by asking me if I would teach an online course. You know who you are.

In writing, or having itself written through me, *Loving to the End … and On* has taught me that it really is the love that matters; all the rest is window dressing. I am grateful.

Endnotes

1 Elizabeth Kübler-Ross, MD, *On Death and Dying* (New York: MacMillan Publishing Co., Inc., 1969) 8.
2 http://www.livescience.com/46993-oldest-medical-report-of-near-death-experience.html
3 http://www.resuscitationjournal.com/article/S0300-9572(14)00588-7/fulltext
4 http://ndestories.org/dr-mary-neal/
5 www.iands.org
6 www.aciste.org
7 http://www.salon.com/2012/04/21/near_death_explained/
8 Melvin Morse, MD with Paul Perry, Parting Visions, Uses and Meanings of Pre-Death, Psychic, and Spiritual Experiences, (New York:Villard Books, 1994)163-64; 170.
9 Pamela M. Kircher, M.D., Love is the Link, A Hospice Doctor Shares Her Experience of Near-Death and Dying(Burdett, N.Y: Larson Publications, 1995) 43.
10 Michael Sabom, MD, *Light and Death* (Grand Rapids, MI: Zondervan Publishing House,1998)14.
11 http://iands.org/about-ndes/common-aftereffects.html
12 https://www.monroeinstitute.org/
13 http://iands.org/about-ndes/nde-and-the-terminally-ill.html
14 Joel L. Whitton, MD, PhD, and Joe Fisher, *Life Between Life* (NYC: Warner Books, 1986)11.
15 http://afterlifeawareness.com
16 Kagan, Annie, The Afterlife of Billy Fingers, How My Bad-Boy Brother Proved to Me There's Life After Death, (Charlottesville, VA: Hampton Roads Publishing Co., Inc., 2013).
17 http://www.arthurfindlaycollege.org/intro/aboutuk.html

18 Michael Murphy and Rhea A. White, *The Psychic Side of Sports*, (Reading, MA:Addison-Wesley Publishing Company, 1978) 62-63.
19 Whitney S Hibbard, Raymond W Worring, and Richard Brennan, *Psychic Criminology, A Guide for Using Psychics in Investigations, Second Edition*, (Springfield, IL: Charles C. Thomas Publisher, Ltd., 2002) 124.
20 Janet Wehr, RN, Peaceful Passages, A Hospice Nurse's Stories of Dying Well, (Wheaton, IL.: Quest Books, 2015) 129.
21 Maggie Callanan and Patricia Kelley, *Final Gifts* (New York: Bantam Books, 1992) 83.
22 http://ajh.sagepub.com/content/23/1/17.abstract
23 Karen M. Wyatt, MD, What Really Matters, 7 Lessons for Living from the Stories of the Dying (NYC: Sunroom Studios, 2011) 7.
24 Marilyn A. Mendoza, PhD, We Do Not Die Alone: "Jesus is Coming to Get Me in a White Pickup Truck" (Dahlonaga, GA: ICAN Publishing Inc., 2008) 21, 27, & 30.
25 Elizabeth Kübler-Ross, MD, On Life After Death (Berkeley,CA: Celestial Arts, 1991) 54.
26 Allen J. Hamilton, MD, FACS. The Scalpel and the Soul, Encounters with Surgery, the Supernatural, and the Healing Power of Hope (New York:Jeremy P. Tarcher/Putnam, 2008) 70-78.
27 http://womenshistory.about.com/od/quotes/a/anna_pavlova.htm
28 Mendoza, *We Do Not Die Alone*, 31.
29 Wehr, Peaceful Passages, 125.
30 Kircher,, Love is the Link, 74.
31 "Deathbed Visions: Hospice Nurses Share Their Stories," https://www.youtube.com/watch?v=nMr_sapd-qY
32 Callanan and Kelley, *Final Gifts*, 96-97.
33 http://www.sharedcrossing.com/shared-death-experience.html
34 W Dewi Rees,"The Hallucinations of Widowhood," *British Medical Journal*, vol. 4 (5778, (Oct.2,1971): 37-41; P.R. Olson, J.A. Suddeth, P.J. Peterson, and C. Egelhoff, "The Hallucinations of Widowhood," *Journal of the American Geriatrics Society*, 33(8) (August 1985): 543-7.
35 http://www.academia.edu/1625789/A New Model of Grief from the English-Speaking World, Dennis Klass, Ph.D.
36 Matt Hendrickson, "Country Queen" *Garden and Gun* (April/May 2016): 41.
37 https://www.youtube.com/watch?v=O7rxKMHL26w
38 Peggy Noonan, "Farewell to Nancy Reagan, A Friend and Patriot, Declarations," *The Wall Street Journal*, (Saturday/Sunday, March 12-13, 2016): A11.

39 *Union Prayer Book, Newly Revised Edition,* Part II, The Central Conference of American Rabbis, (Cincinnati 1945) 90.

40 Raymond Moody, MD, PhD and Paul Perry, Glimpses of Eternity: Sharing of a Loved One's Passage from This Life to the Next, (New York: Guideposts, 2010) chapter 1,

41 http://www.sharedcrossing.com/shared-death-experience.html

42 Julie Bain, *The Rotarian,* vol. 194, no. 6, (Dec. 2015): pp 42-47.

43 Wehr, Peaceful Passages, 157.

44 E. Wesley Ely, MD, "A Swimming Pool in the ICU?" *Wall Street Journal,* (June 17, 2016): A9.

45 Laura Landro, "How to Talk to Your Nurse," *Wall Street Journal,* (July 5, 2016): D1-D2.

46 *HBDI®, Whole Brain® Thinking, Herrmann Brain Dominance Instrument® and Whole Brain® Model* are trademarks and registered trademarks of Herrmann Global LLC. and are registered in the U.S. Patent and Trademark Office. Text and graphics, including graphical trademarks such as the Whole Brain® graph and color scheme, are copyrighted material of Herrmann Global LLC. No part of these printed or electronic materials may be reproduced or utilized in any form or by any means, electronic or mechanical, including photocopying, recording or any information storage and retrieval system without prior written agreement from Herrmann Global, LLC. ©2017 Herrmann Global, LLC

47 *HBDI®, Whole Brain® Thinking, Herrmann Brain Dominance Instrument® and Whole Brain® Model* are trademarks and registered trademarks of Herrmann Global LLC. and are registered in the U.S. Patent and Trademark Office. Text and graphics, including graphical trademarks such as the Whole Brain® graph and color scheme, are copyrighted material of Herrmann Global LLC. No part of these printed or electronic materials may be reproduced or utilized in any form or by any means, electronic or mechanical, including photocopying, recording or any information storage and retrieval system without prior written agreement from Herrmann Global, LLC. ©2017 Herrmann Global, LLC

48 Whole Brain® is a registered trademark of Herrmann Global LLC. Registered in the U.S. Patent and Trademark Office. "HBDI® is a registered trademark of Herrmann Global, LLC." The four-color, four-quadrant graphic is a registered trademark of Herrmann Global, LLC." *HBDI®, Whole Brain® Thinking, Herrmann Brain Dominance Instrument® and Whole Brain® Model* are trademarks and registered trademarks of Herrmann Global, LLC. Text and graphics, including graphical trademarks such as the Whole Brain® graph and color scheme, are copyrighted material of Herrmann Global LLC. No part

of these printed or electronic materials may be reproduced or utilized in any form or by any means, electronic or mechanical, including photocopying, recording or any information storage and retrieval system without prior written agreement from Herrmann Global, LLC. ©2017 Herrmann Global, LLC

49 Whole Brain® is a registered trademark of Herrmann Global LLC. Registered in the U.S. Patent and Trademark Office. "HBDI® is a registered trademark of Herrmann Global, LLC." The four-color, four-quadrant graphic is a registered trademark of Herrmann Global, LLC." *HBDI®, Whole Brain® Thinking, Herrmann Brain Dominance Instrument® and Whole Brain® Model* are trademarks and registered trademarks of Herrmann Global, LLC. Text and graphics, including graphical trademarks such as the Whole Brain® graph and color scheme, are copyrighted material of Herrmann Global LLC. No part of these printed or electronic materials may be reproduced or utilized in any form or by any means, electronic or mechanical, including photocopying, recording or any information storage and retrieval system without prior written agreement from Herrmann Global, LLC. ©2017 Herrmann Global, LLC

50 Our Four Different Selves http://www.herrmannsolutions.com/blog/portfolio-item/creative-and-strategic- thinking-the-coming-competencies/

51 *HBDI®, Whole Brain® Thinking, Herrmann Brain Dominance Instrument® and Whole Brain® Model* are trademarks and registered trademarks of Herrmann Global, LLC., and are registered in the U.S. Patent and Trademark Office. Text and graphics, including graphical trademarks such as the Whole Brain® graph and color scheme, are copyrighted material of Herrmann Global LLC. No part of these printed or electronic materials may be reproduced or utilized in any form or by any means, electronic or mechanical, including photocopying, recording or any information storage and retrieval system without prior written agreement from Herrmann Global, LLC. ©2017 Herrmann Global, LLC

52 HBDI® is a registered trademark of Herrmann Global, LLC.", "Whole Brain® is a registered trademark of Herrmann Global, LLC

53 Ned Herrmann and Ann Herrmann-Nehdi, The Whole Brain Business Book, Unlocking The Power of Whole Brain Thinking in Organizations and Individuals (New York:McGraw Hill, 2015).

54 HBDI®, Whole Brain® Thinking, Herrmann Brain Dominance Instrument® and Whole Brain® Model are trademarks and registered trademarks of Herrmann Global, LLC., and are registered in the U.S. Patent and Trademark Office. Text and graphics, including graphical

trademarks such as the Whole Brain® graph and color scheme, are copyrighted material of Herrmann Global LLC. No part of these printed or electronic materials may be reproduced or utilized in any form or by any means, electronic or mechanical, including photocopying, recording or any information storage and retrieval system without prior written agreement from Herrmann Global, LLC. ©2017 Herrmann Global, LLC

55 Whole Brain® is a registered trademark of Herrmann Global, LLC. Registered in the U.S. Patent and Trademark Office. "HBDI® is a registered trademark of Herrmann Global, LLC." The four-color, four-quadrant graphic is a registered trademark of Herrmann Global, LLC." *HBDI®, Whole Brain® Thinking, Herrmann Brain Dominance Instrument® and Whole Brain® Model* are trademarks and registered trademarks of Herrmann Global, LLC. Text and graphics, including graphical trademarks such as the Whole Brain® graph and color scheme, are copyrighted material of Herrmann Global LLC. No part of these printed or electronic materials may be reproduced or utilized in any form or by any means, electronic or mechanical, including photocopying, recording or any information storage and retrieval system without prior written agreement from Herrmann Global, LLC. ©2017 Herrmann Global, LLC

56 HBDI® Profile on Herrmann International's website: http://www.herrmannsolutions.com/assessment-tools-and- solutions/

57 Whole Brain® is a registered trademark of Herrmann Global, LLC. Registered in the U.S. Patent and Trademark Office. "HBDI® is a registered trademark of Herrmann Global, LLC." The four-color, four-quadrant graphic is a registered trademark of Herrmann Global, LLC." *HBDI®, Whole Brain® Thinking, Herrmann Brain Dominance Instrument® and Whole Brain® Model* are trademarks and registered trademarks of Herrmann Global, LLC. Text and graphics, including graphical trademarks such as the Whole Brain® graph and color scheme, are copyrighted material of Herrmann Global LLC. No part of these printed or electronic materials may be reproduced or utilized in any form or by any means, electronic or mechanical, including photocopying, recording or any information storage and retrieval system without prior written agreement from Herrmann Global, LLC. ©2017 Herrmann Global, LLC

58 Case Study, 1,100 bed hospital http://www.herrmannsolutions.com/blog/portfolio-item/reaching-breakthrough- results/

59 HBDI®, Whole Brain® Thinking, Herrmann Brain Dominance Instrument® and Whole Brain® Model are trademarks and registered trademarks of Herrmann Global, LLC., and are registered in the U.S. Patent and Trademark Office. Text and graphics, including graphical trademarks such as the Whole Brain® graph and color scheme, are copyrighted material of Herrmann Global LLC. No part of these printed or electronic materials may be reproduced or utilized in any form or by any means, electronic or mechanical, including photocopying, recording or any information storage and retrieval system without prior written agreement from Herrmann Global, LLC. ©2017 Herrmann Global, LLC

60 *HBDI®, Whole Brain® Thinking, Herrmann Brain Dominance Instrument® and Whole Brain® Model* are trademarks and registered trademarks of Herrmann Global, LLC., and are registered in the U.S. Patent and Trademark Office. Text and graphics, including graphical trademarks such as the Whole Brain® graph and color scheme, are copyrighted material of Herrmann Global LLC. No part of these printed or electronic materials may be reproduced or utilized in any form or by any means, electronic or mechanical, including photocopying, recording or any information storage and retrieval system without prior written agreement from Herrmann Global, LLC. ©2017 Herrmann Global, LLC

61 Katy Butler, *Knocking on Heaven's Door, The Path To a Better Way of Death* (New York:Scribner, 2013)

62 Sarah Knapton, "Bright Flash of Light Marks Incredible Moment Life Begins When Sperm Meets Egg" *The Telegraph* (April 26,2016): http://www.telegraph.co.uk/science/2016/04/26/bright-flash-of-light- marks-incredible-moment-life-begins-when-s/

63 Janusz Slawinski, ScD, "Electromagnetic Radiation and the Afterlife," *Journal of Near Death Studies,* vol. 6, no. 2 (Winter 1987): http://newdualism.org/nde-papers/Slawinski/Slawinski-Journal%20of%20Near- Death%20Studies_1987-6-79-94.pdf

64 William Joseph Bray, Quantum Physics, Near Death Experiences, Eternal Consciousness, Religion, and the Human Soul (San Bernadino, CA: CreateSpace Independent Publishing Platform, 2012).

Bibliography

Books

Bray, William Joseph, *Quantum Physics, Near Death Experiences, Eternal Consciousness, Religion, and the Human Soul,* San Bernadino, CA: Create Space Independent Publishing Platform, 2012

Butler,Katy, *Knocking on Heaven's Door, The Path to a Better Way of Death,* New York: Scribner, 2013

Callanan, Maggie and Kelley, Patricia, *Final Gifts,* New York: Bantam Books, 1992

Hamilton, Allan J., MD, FACS, *The Scalpel and the Soul, Encounters with Surgery, the Supernatural, and the Healing Power of Hope,* New York: Jeremy P. Tarcher/Putnam, 2008

Herrmann, Ned and Herrmann-Nehdi, Ann, *the Whole Brain Business Book, Unlocking the Power of Whole Brain Thinking in Organizations and Individuals,* New York: McGraw Hill,2015

Hubbard, Whitney S., Worring, Raymond W., and Brennan, Richard, *Psychic Criminology, A Guide for Using Psychics in Investigations, Second Edition,* Springfield, IL: Charles C. Thomas Publisher Ltd., 2002

Kagan, Annie, *The Afterlife of Billy Fingers, How My Bad-Boy Brother Proved to Me There's Life After Death,* Charlottesville, Va: Hampton Roads Publishing Co. Inc., 2013

Kircher, Pamela M., MD, *Love is the Link, A Hospice Doctor Shares Her Experience of Near-Death and Dying*, Burdett, N.Y.: Larson Publications, 1995

Kubler-Ross, Elizabeth, MD, *On Death and Dying,* New York: MacMillan Publishing Co., Inc., 1969

Kubler-Ross, Elizabeth, MD, *On Life After Death,* Berkeley, CA: Celestial Arts, 1991

Mendoza, Marilyn A.,PhD, *We Do Not Die Alone:"Jesus is Coming to Get Me in a White Pickup Truck,"* Dahlonaga, Ga.:ICAN Publishing, 2008

Moody, Raymond, MD,PhD and Perry, Paul, *Glimpses of Eternity: Sharing of a Loved One's*

Passage from This Life to the Next, New York: Guideposts, 2010

Morse, Melvin, MD with Perry, Paul, *Parting Visions, Uses and Meanings of Pre-Death,Psychic, and Spiritual Experiences,* New York:Villard Books, 1994

Murphy, Michael and White, Rhea A., *The Psychic Side of Sports,* Reading, MA, Addison-Wesley Publishing Company, 1978.

Sabom, Michael, MD, *Light and Death,* Grand Rapids, MI: Zondervan Publishing House, 1998

The Central Conference of American Rabbis, *Union Prayerbook,* Cincinnati, Ohio, 1945

Wehr, Janet, RN, *Peaceful Passages, A Hospice Nurse's Stories of Dying Well,* Wheaton, IL: Quest Books, 2015

Whitton, Joel L., MD, PhD, and Fisher, Joe, *Life Between Life,* New York City: Warner Books, 1986

Wyatt, Karen M., MD, *What Really Matters, 7 Lessons fro Living from the Stories of the Dying,* New York: 2011

Journals, Newspapers and Magazines

Bain, Julie. "An Entrepreneur and a Gentleman." *The Rotarian,* vol 194 (6). December, 2015. 42-47.

Ely, E.Wesley. "A Swimming Pool in the ICU?" *Wall Street Journal.* June 17, 2016. A9.

Greyson, B. "Near-death encounters with and without near-death experiences: comparative NDE scale profiles." *Journal of Near Death Studies.* 1990 (8). 151–161.

Hendrickson, Matt. "Interview with Loretta Lynn." *Garden and Gun.* April/May 2016. 41. (Also: http://gardenandgun.com/articles/gg-interview-loretta-lynn/)

Landro, Laura. "How to Talk to Your Nurse." *Wall Street Journal.* July 5, 2016. D1-D2.

Noonan, Peggy. "Farewell to Nancy Reagan, A Friend and Patriot, Declarations." *Wall*

Street Journal. March 12-13, 2016. A11.

Rees, W. Dewi. "The Hallucination of Widowhood." *British Medical Journal,* vol. 4 (5778).

October 2, 1971. 37-41; Olson, P.R., Suddeth, J.A., Peterson, P.J., and Egelhoff, C. "The Hallucination of Widowhood." *Journal of the American Geriatrics Society,* 33(8). August, 1985. 543-7.

Electronic Sources (Web Publications)

Organizations

American Center for the Integration of Spiritually Transformative Experiences, April 2018, https://aciste.org

Arthur Findlay College, April 2018, https://www.arthurfindlaycollege.org https://www.arthurfindlaycollege.org/the-college/ https://www.arthurfindlaycollege.org/find-the-arthur-findlay-college/

HBDI, Herrman Global, LLC, April 2018, https://www.herrmannsolutions.com/herrmann-international/
https://www.herrmannsolutions.com/blog/portfolio-item/creative-and-strategic-thinking-the-coming-competencies/
https://www.herrmannsolutions.com/assessment-tools-and-solutions/
http://www.herrmannsolutions.com/blog/portfolio-item/reaching-breakthrough-results/

International Association of Near Death Studies, April 2018, https://www.iands.org
https://www.iands.org/ndes/about-ndes/what-is-an-nde.html
https://www.iands.org/ndes/about-ndes/common-aftereffects.html
https://www.iands.org/ndes/about-ndes/nde-and-the-terminally-ill.html

Monroe Institute, April 2018, https://www.monroeinstitute.org for April of 2018, Near Death Experience Intensive https://www.monroeinstitute.org/node/3281

The Original Afterlife Awareness Conference, April 2018, https://afterlifeconference.com (formerly afterlifeawareness.com) https://afterlifeconference.com/about-the-afterlife-conference/continuation-of-consciousness-after-death/(who we are)

Shared Crossing Project, April 2018, http://www.sharedcrossing.com http://www.sharedcrossing.com/shared-death-experience.html

Articles

Beauregard, Mario. Salon. April 21, 2012. "Near death, explained." https://www.salon.com/2012/04/21/near_death_explained/

Brayne,Sue,MA, Farnham,Chris,MD, FRCPsych, Fenwick,Peter, MD, FRCPsych. American Journal of Hospice and Palliative Medicine. 2006. "Deathbed phenomena and their effect on a palliative care team: A pilot study." http://journals.sagepub.com/doi/abs/10.1177/104990910602300104

Charlier, Phillippe. Resuscitation Journal. 2014. "Oldest medical description of a near death experience (NDE), France, 18th century" http://www.resuscitationjournal.com/article/S0300-9572%2814%2900588-7/references

Gholipour, Bahar. Live Science. July 24, 2014. https://www.livescience.com/46993-oldest-medical-report-of-near-death-experience.html

Klass, Dennis,PhD. Academia Edu. "A New Model of Grief for the Englilsh-Speaking World." http://www.academia.edu/1625789/A_New_Model_of_Grief_from_the_English-Speaking_World

Knapton, Sarah. "Bright flash of light marks incredible moment life begins when sperm meets egg." April 26, 2016. https://www.telegraph.co.uk//science/2016/04/26/bright-flash-of-light-marks-incredible-moment-life-begins-when-s/

Lewis, Jone Johnson. Anna Pavlova Quotes/Thought Co. March 2017. "Anna Pavlova 1881-1931" https://www.thoughtco.com/anna-pavlova-quotes-3530029

Neal, Mary, MD, http://ndestories.org/dr-mary-neal/

Slawinski, Janusz, ScD, "Electromagnetic Radiation and the Afterlife."

Journal of Near-Death Studies, 6(2) Winter 1987. http://newdualism.org/nde-papers/Slawinski/Slawinski-Journal%20of%20Near-Death%20Studies_1987-6-79-94.pdf

Videos

Deathbed Visions-Hospice Nurses Share Their Stories. NDE Accounts. April 13, 2014. https://www.youtube.com/watch?v=nMr_sapd-qY

Loretta Lynn's Haunted Plantation. Jan.1, 2016. https://www.youtube.com/watch?v=O7rxKMHL26w

